Meal Prep Cookbook for Weight Loss

The Complete Meal Prepping Guide For Beginners to Lose Fat Fast, Reverse Your Bad Health Condition and Live Happily (LOSE 1 POUND PER DAY)

By Tommy C. Mitchell

Contents

INTRODUCTION..7

CHAPTER 1: EVERYTHING ABOUT FAT LOSS MEAL PLAN..8

WHAT IS MEAL PREP?...8

BENEFITS OF MEAL PREP...8

UTENSILS FOR MEAL PREP..8

TIPS AND FAQs...9

GENERAL FOOD GUIDE FOR WEIGHT LOSS...9

CARBOHYDRATES..9

TIPS TO EAT CARBS WITHOUT STOCKING MUCH FAT..9

PROTEINS..10

VITAMINS AND MINERALS...11

APPROPRIATE VITAMIN AND MINERAL INTAKE...11

WATER..11

SUPER FOODS FOE TRIGGERING WEIGHT LOSS..12

EASY MISTAKES TO AVOID..13

CHAPTER 2: MEAL PREP FOR BREAKFAST..14

1.Breakfast Burrito...14

2.Pancakes..15

3.Tropical Smoothie...16

4.Avocado Smoothie...17

5.Parsley Smoothie...18

6.Poblano Tofu Scramble...19

7.Ginger Apple Muffins..20

8.Paleo Quinoa...21

9.Scrambled Tofu..22

10.Scrambled Eggs with Tomatoes..23

11.Chocolate Chunk Banana Bread..24

12.Coconut Flour Pancakes..25

13.Sweet Potato Muffins...26

14.Blueberry Coconut French Toast...27

15.Breakfast Casserole..28

16.Tropical Sunrise Smoothie... 29

17.Pumpkin Smoothie.. 30

18.Crunchy Homemade Granola... 31

CHAPTER 3: MEAL PREP FOR LUNCH... **32**

19.Kale, Beet, Salmon Salad.. 32

20.Garlic Shrimp...33

21.Hot & Spicy Sweet Potato Salad..34

22.Roasted Sweet Potatoes & Black Bean Burrito.. 35

23.Black & White Bean, Sweet Potato Soup...36

24.Collard Greens... 37

25.Lentil Soup... 38

26.Broccoli, Carrots, Peas, and Chard Stir Fry..39

27.Cauliflower Rice Stir Fry.. 40

28.Boiled Fowl with Rice.. 41

29.Vegan Spaghetti with Anchovies..42

30.Spicy Chard with Tofu...43

31.Polenta & Beans Mix... 44

32.Vegan Split Pea & Sweet Potato Soup... 45

33.Taco Salad In A Mason jar...46

34.Lettuce Tacos with Chipotle Chicken.. 47

35.Spicy Picadillo Lettuce Wrap...48

36.California Turkey, Bacon Lettuce Wrap with Basil Mayo................................ 49

37.Steak with Siracha Lettuce Wrap... 50

38.Cajun Shrimp Noodle Bowl.. 51

39.Egg Roll In A Bowl.. 52

40.Anti-Pasto Salad..53

CHAPTER 4: MEAL PREP FOR DINNER.. **54**

41.Rabbit with Mustard.. 54

42.Vegan Tofu Vegetable Stir Fry..55

43.Paleo Chickpeas with Cumin.. 56

44.Grilled Swordfish with Herbs...57

45.Fish Fillets with Sesame...58

46.Chickpea Soup...59

47.Fresh Salmon with Vegetables...60

48.Quinoa with Vegetables..61

49.Grilled Salmon with Peppers...62

50.Skillet Chicken Thighs With Butternut Squash.................................63

51.Sweet Potato Turkey Casserole W/Eggplant and Tomato..........................64

52.Paleo Pizza Soup..65

53.Spicy Pumpkin Chili...66

54.Creamy Basil And Tomato Chicken...67

55.Amazing Ground Turkey and Spinach Stuffed Mushroom..........................68

56.Shepherd's Pie with Cauliflower Topping...69

57.Sweet and Sour Pork Chop...70

CHAPTER 5: MEAL PREP FOR SNACKS..**71**

58.Very Sweet Potatoes...71

59.Pumpkin Soup...72

60.Stuffed Mushrooms...73

61.Lean Green Smoothie..74

Fiber: 3.8g62.Candied Pecans...74

63.Balsamic Rosemary Roasted Vegetables...76

64.Spiced and Crispy Carrot Chips...77

65.Eggplant Caponata..78

66.Sautéed Mushrooms..79

67.Sautéed Radishes..80

68.Roasted Heirloom Carrots...81

69.Beans With Crushed Almonds..82

70.Cauliflower Couscous with Apricots and Cashews.............................83

CHAPTER 6: MEAL PREP FOR SWEET TREATS..................................**84**

71.Flourless Chocolate Cake..84

72.Biscotti with Almonds...85

73.Strawberry Yogurt Cornflake Parfait..86

74.Choco Berry Mousse...87

75. Strawberry Frozen Yogurt...88

76. Avocado Smoothie..89

77. Raspberry-Peach Crumble...90

78. Fresh Strawberry Parfait..91

79. Beets & Berries Smoothie...92

80. Strawberry Cheesecake...93

81. Fruit Granita..94

82. Graham Crackers...95

83. Mango Chia Seed Pudding..96

84. Chocolaty Cocoa Mousse...97

85. Pumpkin Nut Butter Cup...98

86. Chocolate Silk Pie...99

87. Cinnamon Apple Chips...100

88. Blueberry Smoothie...101

Conclusion...102

Have you ever wondered what social-economic and health effects are associated with being overweight? Gaining a few pounds in a year may not seem problematic. But an uncontrolled accumulation of pounds over time can lead to detrimental health and social-economic effects. Mainly, being overweight can cause various health problems, including cardiovascular diseases, fatty liver disease, high blood pressure, osteoarthritis, and even sleep apnea.

But now you will have a good solution for your overweight! With this amazing Meal Prep Cookbook, you will easily cut your weight in few weeks. All you need to do is just to follow it and put it into action!

This meal prep cookbook is your answer to fully understanding how to fuel your body so you can burn fat 24/7. It is a complete meal prep guide leading you to HOW, WHAT, and WHEN to prep. You will learn everything about meal prep for rapid weight loss, heal your body and have a better lifestyle.

We have prepared with 88 delicious and easy recipes, including: breakfasts, lunches, dinners, sweet treats and snacks that are tasty, delicious. Meantime all recipes include all the macros to make tracking simple. You can find **meat, vegetables, smoothies, noodles, beef, and pork** among the delicious and healthy recipes.With the detailed step by step procedure for each recipe, even the non-cook can prepare these recipes quickly and easily!

Having the macros counted will simplify your life. You will always have an idea of your caloric intake and customize them to your requirements. Most of the recipes can be made in 20 minutes, sometimes less. It will save you too much time! With this amazing fat loss meal prep book, you will achieve incredible effects. In the next few weeks you will be surprised when you stand before the mirror.

PLEASE ENJOY IT!

Therefore, you should not eat sugar outside dining. You can eat your carbs with a source of fat, protein, or fibrous vegetables that will slow their digestion and regulate the release of sugar into your bloodstream. Also, you can eat only low glycemic foods, which are broken down and digested slowly.

By doing this, you will enjoy the most of your carbohydrates as an energy source and will limit fat storage.

Avoid Carbs that are processed as Fat

When your body energy is excess, and your glycogen stores (muscles and liver) are full, the surplus carbohydrates you eat is turned into fat. The ideal time to consume your carbs is in the morning and around your workouts.

When to eat your Carbs

To avoid running out of carbohydrates or ruin your body and your health because of them, I will now tell you when to eat your carbs. Most people store fat when they eat carbohydrates because they deplete at the wrong time. If you consume your carbohydrates at specific, appropriate times, you will not have to worry about gaining fat.

PROTEINS

Proteins are foods that when consumed, help in building the body as well as repairing body tissue. If you want to have a proper looking body then protein is your answer. This includes, legumes, beef, chicken, and milk. Pretty sure you can access at least a few of these foods. So how do proteins aid in weight loss?

Eat high amounts of Protein

High amounts of proteins are healthy when consumed for body building and also for reducing weight. When you consume large quantities of proteins, the rate of metabolism is equally high. This is paramount in ensuring reduction of appetite and, therefore, regulating weight-related hormones. What proteins do to reduce weight is reduce your appetite so eventually your calories levels drop automatically.

Making right Protein choices

I just took you through the necessity of high proteins for weight loss. However, you must not forget that there is a limit beyond which when proteins are considered detrimental to your health. Remember our focus is attaining a healthy body with reduced weight; or you end up focusing on reducing weight and forget that your body should also remain healthy.

Proteins that are best for your health

You are already aware that you should not take extreme levels of proteins. It is, therefore, important to know what proteins are best for your body and which ones should be avoided.

Animal proteins, such as beef, chicken, and fish provide you with amino acid required for optimal protein consumption and healthy eating. This is not to say plant proteins are not also advisable. I am just stating that, if you need high levels of Amino acids, and then feed on animal proteins since plant proteins provide reduced levels of amino acid. Most importantly, you should be careful with processed proteins since they consist, for instance, embedded salts that could result in increased blood pressure levels. Therefore, know what proteins to consume, in what amounts to ensure you maintain your goal of weight loss while remaining healthy.

Vitamins and minerals are compounds that are organic and usually consumed in small amounts as the body cannot synthesize them. They facilitate proper functioning of the body after consumption of other food components. Examples of foods that provide the body with vitamins and minerals are; carrots, tropical fruits, dark leafy greens, calcium, chromium, and squash.

Best Vitamins for weight control in a healthy manner

Vitamins could be used as a perfect way to keep a healthy body at an ideal weight. Some of these vitamins are discussed below:

(a) Vitamin B12

Vitamin B12 soluble in water and is usually essential in ensuring proper usage of calories in the body, as well as red blood cell creation. This vitamin is found in some animal proteins such as beef, chicken, and fish. Vitamin B12 is necessary for giving the body the required energy to exercise and eventual weight loss.

(b) Fiber

Here is another vitamin that most of us don't pay attention to. Research has shown that taking high amounts of fiber results in reduced appetite, which then means fewer calories are taken in. A person who consumes higher amounts of fiber stands the chance to improve his or her digestion and also an excellent opportunity to lose weight without having to take in any pills.

(c) Chromium

Chromium is a mineral that is necessary for sugar metabolism as well as aiding to maintain proper fat levels. People who consume chromium have been observed to record high levels of weight loss.

APPROPRIATE VITAMIN AND MINERAL INTAKE

So you want to lose weight in a healthy manner? Then mind the vitamin and mineral quantities consumed. Vitamins are in some way meant to supplement the food you take in. You, therefore, should be careful not to make them your primary food. Excess consumption of vitamins and minerals results in over-accumulation in the body especially for the ones that are soluble in fats. Precaution must be taken since too much of it is harmful, and nobody eats to cause harm to their body.

WATER

If you want to be healthy with the best weight possible, then I have what you need; water. Being free from calories, water is the drink to take most often. One should drink at least 1 and a half gallons of water per day.

Water for weight loss

Have you ever realized that you eat less when you drink water before taking your meals? If you have not realized that, then it is high time you tried that out. Drinking water increases the amount of fluids in your body yet you can still use it for appetite loss. That means you will be losing weight but boosting fluid levels in your body. Good strategy, isn't it?

How much water for fit weight loss

You must be thinking that no matter the amount of water taken, it does not matter? Well, that is not the case. Two glasses of water before every meal is enough to reduce appetite. Remember, I am not asking you to suppress your appetite completely. You need to remain healthy, and so you must take appropriate amounts of food. Excessive water becomes a burden to the kidneys to push it out of the body, resulting in waterlogging in the blood. Am sure you do not want that.

SUPER FOODS FOR TRIGGERING WEIGHT LOSS

Weight issues have been a world-wide problem. There are many trying multiple modus-operandi to lose weight in order to get rid of the symptoms associated with extra weight; pain in joints, knees, diabetes, stroke, heart attack, metabolic syndrome, osteoarthritis, cancer, sleep apnea, gallstones, and reproductive problems, amongst other health issues.

We are going to share some information that can be very useful for the person persevering for weight loss.

1. **Apples**

"An apple a day keeps the doctor away." You have probably heard that saying. So eat an apple every day and its phytonutrients, antioxidants, and dietary fiber will keep you slim and fit. You can eat an apple anytime.

2. **Oats**

Carbohydrates found in oats are very useful in terms of releasing hormone serotonin, which burns fat faster than any other thing. Moreover, it provides relaxation. You can add them to any meal.

3. **Yogurt**

Yogurt is one of the most easily digestible in comparison to milk. Calcium and Vitamin-B are one of the most important parts of its properties that are known for boosting immunity. Yogurt is a kind of medicine available in your home that contains probiotics and aids in having a healthy digestive tract which could lead to the prevention of colon cancer. Not to mention it contains calcium, vitamin b-2 and b-12, potassium, and magnesium

4. **Pomegranate**

Pomegranates provide us a high amount of fiber. Moreover, pomegranates are a rich source of antioxidants and folic acid. Pomegranates are fantastic alternative for sugar. Try it and satisfy your sugar cravings.

5. **Lentils**

Lentils are very good source of protein and fiber. In addition, lentils also offer marvelous resistant starch fiber; a kind of carbohydrate that improves our metabolic process and burns unnecessary fat.

6. **Green tea**

Do you drink tea containing caffeine? If your answer is yes, you need to switch to green tea. Switching to green tea 2-3 cups a day not only enhances your fat burning process via antioxidants present in it but also reduces your weight faster.

7. **Watermelon**

Water is the most dominating property of watermelon. It has 92% water and Vitamin A and C, which fuel weight loss naturally. It is wonderful in taste and perfect for quenching your thirst, especially on hot summer days.

These are some of the super foods that you can include in your diet and trigger weight loss. However, it is also strongly recommended you consult a physician before beginning any weight loss regime.

EASY MISTAKES TO AVOID

Some people in the course of losing weight starve themselves and exercise on an empty stomach, or take unnecessary pills amongst other mistakes. This content is meant to highlight these issues in regards to weight loss.

Starving

One easy mistake people make in the course of weight loss program is starving. Starving deprives your body of the right nutrients required to flourish. Eating the right type of food, especially food with high fiber content is very necessary as it burns fat easily. Eating fiber-rich foods prevents eating junkies as it fills your stomach properly.

Breakfast must also not be skipped as skipping it creates the possibility of craving high calorie snacks, which can lead to weight gain and defeating the purpose of weight loss.

Exercising on an empty stomach

Another easy mistake to avoid when following a weight loss plan is exercising on an empty stomach. This is very detrimental to the body. In fact, it is likened to torturing your own body. They body gets harmed while accommodating strenuous activities when you exercise on an empty stomach. Never go for an exercise without taking your meals. This includes hitting the gym. Always eat healthy snacks, such as salads and drink plenty of water or fresh juice to boost your energy.

Pills

Using pills for weight loss is also harmful to the body. It is very tempting for people to want to lose weight fast which leads to taking pills, it is not recommended as these pills contain toxic substances that are harmful to the body on the long run. However, vitamins for weight loss remain a good and viable option as it not harmful to the body since it is natural. If you have to take pills, make sure it is made from natural herbs.

Focusing On Quick Weight Loss

This is another easy mistake. In fact, majority of people fall into this category. Weight loss is never a short term goal, it is long term program. It is well known that people who focus on quick weight loss never achieve good result. Instead of focusing on quick weight loss plan, it is better and rewarding to create a healthy diet plan and also an exercise routine.

Making mistakes in achieving the desired weight loss is common. However, efforts must be made to avoid falling into this trap especially in the area of starving and eating pills as these can cause more harm to the body than good. It is also important to note that weight loss is a long term program.

1.Breakfast Burrito

Prep time: 3 minutes. Cook time: 10 minutes. Servings: 4.

A burrito is a delicious and portable answer to your breakfast.

Ingredients
- 2 soft tortilla wraps
- 4 large eggs
- 2 bunches of spinach
- 1 tomato, diced
- 1 cup sliced mushrooms cut
- 1 garlic clove, minced
- Pinch of salt and pepper
- Coconut oil or oil of your choice.

Preparation

Preheat oven to 300F
1. Wrap soft tortilla shells in foil. Place in oven as you prepare eggs.
2. In a bowl, combine eggs, salt, and pepper. Whisk until combined.
3. In a skillet, heat the oil. Sauté the garlic for 1 minute. Add the mushrooms, tomato. Cook until softened.
4. Pour egg mixture into skillet. Using a spatula, stir continuously as eggs cook. Add spinach. Stir until combined, and wilted.
5. Remove tortilla shells from oven. Set on plates. Fill with egg mixture. Roll, secure with a toothpick. Serve immediately.

Nutrition Value

Calories: 234

Protein: 12g

Fat: 6g

Saturates: 1g

Carbs: 33g

Sugar: 2.5g

Fiber: 1g

2.Pancakes

Prep time: 3 minutes. Cook time: 10 minutes. Servings: 4.

Everybody loves pancakes. Follow this recipe to prepare a new taste.

Ingredients
- 2½ cups all-purpose flour
- 2½ cups of water
- 4 Tbsp granulated sugar
- 2 Tbsp canola oil
- 4 tsp baking powder
- 1 tsp salt

Preparation
1. In a large bowl, combine flour, sugar, baking powder, and salt. Stir gently with whisk until combined.
2. Slowly add water and oil. Stir with spatula until mixed; lumpy mixture is normal.
3. In a large skillet or griddle heat canola oil on medium-high heat.
4. Using ¼ cup measure, ladle batter onto pan. Cook until top is covered with bubbles. Flip and cook for 1-2 minutes. Repeat until batter used up. Serve immediately.

Nutrition Value
Calories: 263
Protein: 4g
Fat: 3g
Saturates: 1g
Carbs: 55g
Sugar: 8g
Fiber: 1g

3. Tropical Smoothie

Prep time: 5 minutes. Servings: 4.

Delicious tropical green smoothie is packed with nutrients in every sip.

Ingredients

- 1 cup coconut water
- ½ cup pumpkin puree
- 1 frozen banana
- 1 Tbsp stevia
- 1 cup baby spinach
- 1 Tbsp ultimate Paleo powder
- 1 Tbsp chia seeds
- ¾ cup fresh mango chunks
- 1 cup ice cubes

Directions

1. Place all ingredients in a blender.
2. Blend until smooth. Serve immediately.

Nutrition Value:

Calories: 244
Protein: 6g
Fat: 4g
Saturates: 1g
Carbs: 50g
Sugar: 32g
Fiber: 10g

4.Avocado Smoothie

Prep time: 5 minutes. Servings: 4.

Avocado smoothie is the perfect meal for a quick breakfast or a snack.

Ingredients

- 1 avocado, diced
- 1 Tbsp ultimate Paleo powder
- 1 Tbsp Coconut oil
- I Tbsp Xylitol
- 1 Tbsp chia seeds
- 1 tsp expresso
- ½ Tbsp raw cacao
- ⅓ cup coconut milk

Directions

1. Place all ingredients in to a blender.
2. Blend until smooth. Serve immediately.

Nutrition Value:

Calories: 433
Protein: 9.8g
Fat: 23.8g
Saturates: 6.8g
Carbs: 45.7g
Sugar: 23.8g
Fiber: 10.2g

5.Parsley Smoothie

Prep time: 5 minutes. Servings: 4

If your main goal is to lose weight, you will never go wrong with this smoothie.

Ingredients

- 1 small bunch fresh parsley, rough chopped
- 1 Tbsp arrowroot powder
- ½ avocado, diced
- 1 pear, peeled, diced
- 2 plums, peeled, diced
- 1 Royal Gala apple, peeled, diced
- 6 medium bananas, peeled, diced
- 1 apple, peeled, diced
- 1 cup of ice
- 1 cup of water

Directions

1. Place all ingredients into a blender.
2. Blend until smooth. Enjoy.

Nutrition Value:

Calories: 413
Protein: 6.8g
Fat: 21.2g
Saturates: 6g
Carbs: 40.7g
Sugar: 20g
Fiber: 13g

6.Poblano Tofu Scramble

Prep time: 3 minutes. Cook time: 10 minutes. Servings: 4.

A meal ideal for people aiming at losing some pounds.

Ingredients
- 1 x 16oz package water-packed tofu
- 1 Tbsp olive oil
- 1 poblano pepper, seeded, chopped
- 2 garlic cloves, minced
- 1 small onion, chopped
- 2 tomatoes, seeded, diced
- ½ tsp dried oregano, crushed
- 1 tsp chili powder
- ½-tsp ground cumin
- 1 Tbsp lime juice
- ¼ tsp salt

Directions
1. Drain the tofu, cut in half. Pat each half with paper towels until dry. Crush tofu in a bowl. Set aside.
2. Heat olive oil in a medium skillet over low-high heat. Sauté garlic, onion, and pepper. Cook for 3 minutes while stirring.
3. Add oregano, chili powder, cumin, and salt. Cook for 1 minute.
4. Add crushed tofu to pan, lower the heat. Cook 4-6 minutes.
5. Drizzle lime juice. Add the tomatoes. Stir to combine.

Nutrition Value
Calories: 182
Protein: 13g
Fat: 9g
Saturates: 1g
Carbs: 11g
Sugar: 59g
Fiber: 3g

7.Ginger Apple Muffins

Prep time: 5 minutes. Cook time: 15-25 minutes. Servings: 4.

For a perfect breakfast idea, try the ginger apple muffin for excellent results.

Ingredients

- 2 cups all-purpose flour
- ⅔ cup granulated sugar, or sugar-substitute
- 1 Tbsp of baking powder
- ½ tsp of salt
- 1 tsp ground cinnamon
- 1 tsp of ground ginger
- ¾ cup unsweetened almond milk
- 1 cup shredded apple
- ½ cup ripe banana, mashed
- 1 Tbsp apple cider vinegar
- ½ cup crystallized ginger (finely chopped)

Preparations

Preheat oven to 400°F

1. Lightly grease a muffin tin, or line with paper liners.
2. In a medium bowl, blend together flour, sugar, baking powder, salt, cinnamon, and ginger.
3. In a separate bowl, mix milk, apple, banana, and vinegar. Stir until combined.
4. Add the dry ingredients to the wet. Stir until combined. Will be lumpy.
5. Fill your muffin cups to ⅔ full.
6. Bake 15 minutes. Insert toothpick in center, if it comes out clean, muffins are done. Continue cooking, check after 5 minute intervals.
7. Allow to cool before removing from pan.

Nutrition Value

Calories: 234
Protein: 12g
Fat: 6g
Saturates: 1g
Carbs: 33g
Sugar: 2.5g
Fiber: 1g

8.Paleo Quinoa

Prep time: 5 minutes. Cook time: 25 minutes. Servings: 4.

Quinoa is the gluten-free wonder grain we can never get enough of.

Ingredients
- 8 oz. quinoa seeds
- Water

Preparation
1. Rinse the seeds of quinoa to remove residue of saponin.
2. In a saucepan, add the quinoa and twice its volume of water.
3. Bring to a boil, turn down heat.
4. Cook covered over low heat until water absorbed, approximately 10 to 15 minutes.
5. Remove from heat. Leave covered another 10 minutes.
6. Using a fork, fluff the quinoa. Serve.

Nutrition Value
Calories: 190
Protein: 6g
Fat: 3g
Saturates: 2g
Carbs: 34g
Sugar: 2g
Fiber: 1g

9.Scrambled Tofu

Prep time: 5 minutes. Cook time: 30 minutes. Servings: 3.

Packed with vegetables and tastes great.

Ingredients

- 1 pound tofu, diced, dried
- 6 Tbsp dry yeast
- ½ tsp garlic powder
- 2 Tbsp tamari
- ½ tsp turmeric
- ½ tsp onion powder
- ½ cup sunflower seeds
- ½ tsp sea salt
- 1 yellow onion
- 2 Tbsp extra-virgin olive oil
- 4 green onions
- 3 garlic cloves, minced
- 1 red bell pepper
- 10 asparagus, break off stems

Directions

1. Mash the tofu in a large bowl. A garlic, onion, and tamari, yeast, salt, and turmeric. Stir until combined.
2. Heat oil in a large skillet on medium high. Pour in sunflower seeds. Cook the seeds for 3 to 4 minutes, frequently stirring the whole time.
3. Stir in the green onion, yellow onion, garlic, and bell pepper. Cover. Steam for 8 minutes.
4. When done, push vegetables to the side. Add tofu to pan.
5. Place vegetables on top of tofu. Add the asparagus on top.
6. Cover and cook on medium 10 to 16 minutes. Flip when brown.
7. Dish is ready when asparagus are fork tender.

Nutrition Value

Calories: 252

Protein: 12g

Fat: 19g

Saturates: 3g

Carbs: 12.7g

Sugar: 2.5g

Fiber: 3g

10.Scrambled Eggs with Tomatoes

Prep time: 3 minutes. Cook time: 7 minutes. Servings: 4.

Variety of greens, tomatoes, and peppers combined with eggs can absolutely make a great start to the day.

Ingredients
- 8 eggs
- 1 tsp olive oil
- ½ cup onion, chopped
- ½ cup tomatoes, seeded, chopped
- ¼ cup green sweet pepper, chopped
- ¼ cup fat-free milk
- ⅛ tsp black pepper, ground
- ¼ tsp salt

Directions
1. In a large skillet, heat olive oil over low-medium heat.
2. Sauté sweet pepper and onion 4 minutes. Stir in the tomato.
3. In a separate bowl, beat eggs, milk, black pepper, and salt together. Add to the skillet. Stir.
4. Using a rubber spatula, stir continuously until eggs cooked. Serve.

Nutrition Value
Calories: 114
Protein: 13g
Fat: 4g
Saturates: 1g
Carbs: 33g
Sugar: 7g
Fiber: 1g

11. Chocolate Chunk Banana Bread

(Prep time: 10 minutes\ Cook time: 50 minutes| 10 servings)

While it is true that Banana bread is really cool, you can't go wrong with banana bread dipped in chocolate! Simple yet elegant recipe will help you start off your day with a burst of chocolaty goodness and a healthy aura.

Ingredients:

- 4 medium Bananas, mashed
- 4 eggs
- ½ cup of almond butter
- 4 Tablespoons of melted coconut oil
- ½ cup of coconut flour
- ½ teaspoon of cinnamon
- 1 teaspoon of baking powder
- 1 teaspoon of pure vanilla extract
- Pinch of salt
- 6 ounces dark chocolate, chopped

Preparation:

Preheat oven 350F

1) Grease a 9 x 5 loaf pan.
2) In a large bowl, combine the mashed banana, coconut oil, eggs, pure vanilla extract and nut butter. Stir well.
3) Add the cinnamon, coconut flour, baking soda, sea salt and baking powder. Stir until combined.
4) Pour into greased pan.
5) Bake 40 minutes, for square pan, or 60 minutes for loaf pan.
6) Check center with a tooth pick, remove when it comes out clean.
7) Allow to cool for 30 minutes before removing from pan.

Nutrition Values

- Calories: 250
- Fat: 18.2g
- Carbohydrates: 19.4g
- Protein: 6.8g
- Dietary Fiber: 3.2g

12.Coconut Flour Pancakes

(Prep time: 5 minutes\ Cook time: 5 minutes| 2 servings)

Who doesn't love a healthy stack of pancakes to start the day off? With this recipe, you can have your fill.

Ingredients:

- 2 teaspoons extra virgin coconut oil
- 1 Tablespoon of raw honey
- 3 large eggs
- ¼ cup of coconut milk
- ½ teaspoon of pure vanilla extract
- ¼ cup of coconut flour
- ¼ teaspoon of tartar cream
- ⅛ teaspoon of baking soda
- ⅛ teaspoon of sea salt

Preparation:

Preheat oven to 350F
1) In a large bowl combine all the ingredients.
2) Grease muffin tin with coconut oil or paper liners.
3) Pour batter evenly in the tin.
4) Bake 35 minutes until golden brown.
5) Cool 15 minutes before removing.

Nutrition Values

- Calories: 65
- Fat: 4.2g
- Carbohydrates: 3.6g
- Protein: 2.5g
- Dietary Fiber: 1.1g

13.Sweet Potato Muffins
(Prep time: 10 minutes\ Cook time: 40 minutes| 9 servings)

Were you afraid that going all Paleo you might need to sacrifice cupcakes? Well don't fret. These muffins deliver a delicious punch and your diet won't suffer for it.

Ingredients:

- ¾ cup of mashed sweet potatoes
- ½ cup of shredded carrot
- ½ cup of grated apple
- ½ cup of shredded coconut
- ½ cup of raisins
- ¼ cup of chopped up dried figs
- ½ cup of chopped up walnuts
- ¾ cup of almond flour
- ⅛ cup of maple syrup
- 1 teaspoon of cinnamon
- ⅛ teaspoon of nutmeg
- 1 teaspoon of baking powder
- 2 eggs

Preparation:

1) In a large bowl, mix coconut oil and honey. Mix until combined. Add the eggs one at a time. Stir well.
2) Add the vanilla and coconut milk. Mix well until smooth.
3) Add the coconut flour. Mix until smooth.
4) Once combined, add tartar cream, salt, and baking soda. Mix well.
5) Heat ghee or coconut oil in frying pan on medium heat. Using a ladle, pour small portion of batter in pan. Swirl the mixture until a thin layer covers the bottom of pan.
6) Once bottom is golden brown, flip to other side. Cook until golden brown.
7) Serve hot with maple syrup.

Nutrition Values

- Calories: 100
- Fat: 5g
- Carbohydrates: 10g
- Protein: 6g
- Dietary Fiber: 5g

14.Blueberry Coconut French Toast

(Prep time: 15 minutes\ Cook time: 40 minutes| 8-10 servings)

This French toast is a dreamy delight for those who are looking for something a little bit sweet with bits of crunch and berry goodness.

Ingredients:

- 1 french baguette
- 2.5 cups of coconut milk
- 6 eggs
- 1 teaspoon of cinnamon
- ½ teaspoon of salt
- 1 cup of fresh blueberries
- 1 cup of unsweetened shredded coconut

For the Sauce

- 2 cups of blueberries
- ¾ cup of water
- 1 teaspoon of honey
- 1 Tablespoon of lemon juice

Preparation:

1) Grease a 9 x 13 baking dish.
2) Slice the baguette into one inch slices. Place them in a single layer in the baking dish.
3) In a separate bowl, combine the eggs, salt, milk, and cinnamon. Stir until well combined.
4) Pour mixture over slices of bread. Turn them to coat evenly.
5) Sprinkle some coconut. Marinade in the fridge overnight.
6) When ready to cook, preheat oven to 350F.
7) Add 1 cup of blueberries to the prepared French toast.
8) Bake for 40 minutes, until golden brown.
9) As the french toast cooks, in a small saucepan, combine the ingredients for the blueberry sauce.
10) Gently cook on medium, until desired consistency is achieved.
11) **Once the french toast is cooked, serve on plates, pour the blueberry sauce over french toast.**

Nutrition Values

- Calories: 111
- Fat: 8g
- Carbohydrates: 5g
- Protein: 5.5g
- Dietary Fiber: 3g

15.Breakfast Casserole

(Prep time: 10 minutes\ Cook time: 70 minutes| 6 servings)

Making a perfect casserole can be somewhat of a challenge. But this one has been carefully crafted and outlined to make sure it is successful.

Ingredients:

- 2 large sweet potatoes, washed, peeled, sliced
- ¼ onion, chopped
- 1 garlic clove, minced
- 3 Tablespoons of olive oil
- ¼ cup mushrooms, sliced
- ½ cup Italian sausage
- 10 eggs
- 1 green onion, sliced
- Salt and pepper

Preparation:

1) In a large frying pan, heat up 1 tablespoon of oil. Add the garlic and onion. Sauté until translucent.
2) Add diced sweet potatoes. Add more oil if needed. Cook for 15 minutes, until fork tender.
3) Place potatoes in a thin layer in greased baking dish.
4) Add the sliced mushrooms to the frying pan. Sauté for 2 minutes, until tender. Season with salt and pepper. Place the mushrooms in a thin layer over the potatoes.
5) Next, cook the sausage in the pan. Season with salt and pepper.
6) As the sausage cooks, preheat oven to 350F.
7) In a large bowl, whisk the eggs. Season with salt and pepper. Pour over the layers in the baking dish.
8) Bake the casserole for 70 minutes, until the eggs are no longer runny.
9) Serve hot.

Nutrition Values

- Calories: 287
- Fat: 19g
- Carbohydrates: 13g
- Protein: 16g
- Dietary Fiber: 2g

16.Tropical Sunrise Smoothie

(Prep time: 5 minutes\ Cook time: nil| 1 serving)

Want to maintain a strict diet and remain healthy? Don't look any further. Blend up this smoothie!

Ingredients:

Portion 1

- ½ a frozen banana
- ½ cup of fresh orange juice
- ¾ cup of frozen mango
- ¼ cup of water

Portion 2

- ½ a frozen banana
- ¾ cup of frozen strawberries
- ½ cup of water
- a few ice cubes

Preparation:

1) Blend the first portion of ingredients. Pour into a glass.
2) Quickly blend the ingredients of second portion.
3) Pour half of second portion to portion 1 mixture, mix them together
4) Once an orange pinkish texture has been achieved, very slowly pour the mixture into the cup with portion 1
5) Then add rest of portion 2 mixture. Stir slowly.
6) And you are done. Enjoy!

Nutrition Values

- Calories: 240
- Fat: 8g
- Carbohydrates: 22g
- Protein: 20g
- Dietary Fiber: 6g

17.Pumpkin Smoothie

(Prep time: 3 minutes\ Cook time: nil| 2 servings)

A healthy kick to your morning or afternoon. Whipping this up will give you energy to fulfill all the tasks on your 'to do' list.

Ingredients:

- ½ a ripe banana
- ½ cup of pumpkin puree
- 2 cups of almond milk
- 2 Tablespoons of peanut butter
- 5 ice cubes
- 2 dates
- ⅛ teaspoon of ground ginger
- ¼ teaspoon of cinnamon
- Pinch of nutmeg

Preparation:

1) Add all the ingredients to the blender. Combine until smooth.
2) Serve cold!

Nutrition Values

Calories: 220 Fat: 6.4g Carbohydrates: 38g Protein: 5.6g Dietary Fiber: 6.1g

18.Crunchy Homemade Granola

(Prep time: 10 minutes\ Cook time: 40 minutes| 2 servings)

No more will you need to buy processed granola.

Ingredients:

- 2 cups of raw walnuts
- 2 cups of raw cashew
- 1 cup of raw pumpkin seeds
- ¼ cup oats
- 1 cup of unsweetened shredded coconut
- 1 cup of dried cranberries
- 1 egg white
- 2 Tablespoons of water
- 3 Tablespoons of grapeseed oil
- ⅓ cup of honey
- 1 teaspoon of pure vanilla extract
- ½ teaspoon of ground cinnamon
- ½ teaspoon of kosher salt

Preparation:

Preheat oven to 300F.
1) Line a cookie sheet with parchment paper.
2) Toss first 3 ingredients in food processor. Pulse until chopped.
3) In a large bowl, whisk egg white until fluffy, approximately 2 minutes.
4) Add grape seed oil, pure vanilla extract, honey, cinnamon and pinch of salt to egg white mixture. Whisk until combined.
5) Pour the chopped nuts and oats into the mixture. Stir until evenly coated.
6) Add the cranberries and shredded coconut to mixture. Stir well.
7) Pour the mixture in a thin layer on your cookie sheet.
8) Bake for 30 minutes, until golden brown.
9) Let it rest 10 minutes before eating.
10) Once completely cooled, store in air tight container.

Nutrition Values

- Calories: 265
- Fat: 19.1g
- Carbohydrates: 20.2g
- Protein: 7.4g
- Dietary Fiber: 3.7g

19.Kale, Beet, Salmon Salad

Prep time: 10 minutes. Cook time: 20 minutes. Servings: 4.

Delicious salad and you don't need to be a chef to prepare it.

Ingredients:

- ⅔ cup cider vinegar
- 2 tsp white vinegar
- ½ cup water
- 1 cup red onion sliced
- 3 tsp honey
- 4 golden beets, trimmed
- 2 Tbsp extra virgin olive oil
- Pinch of salt and black pepper
- 1 tsp mustard
- 6 cups curly kale, stemmed
- 1 x 12oz can salmon, skinless, boneless, drained
- ¼ cup almonds, toasted, sliced

Preparation

1. In a small pan, combine ⅔ cup cider vinegar, water, 2 teaspoons of the honey. Stir and bring to a boil.
2. Add onion. Boil 1 minute. Remove from heat. Set aside. After 10 minutes, drain liquid.
3. Wrap beets in parchment paper. Heat in the microwave for 7 minutes.
4. Rub beets with paper towels to remove skin. Cut into wedges. Set aside.
5. In a bowl, combine 2 tablespoons vinegar, 1 teaspoon honey, the oil, mustard, salt, and pepper. Stir well.
6. Add kale and beets. Stir gently. Place on serving plates.
7. Top each serving with salmon mixture. Garnish with almonds. Serve immediately.

Nutrition Value

Calories: 236
Protein: 34g
Fat: 7g
Saturates: 1g
Carbs: 16g
Sugar: 2g
Fiber: 6g

20.Garlic Shrimp

Prep time: 5 minutes. Cook time: 10 minutes. Servings: 2.

Shrimp and garlic, a mouth-watering combo.

Ingredients

- 3 garlic cloves, minced
- 3 Tbsp olive oil
- 1 Tbsp paprika
- 2 Tbsp brandy
- Pinch of salt and pepper
- Fresh basil leaves, rough chopped

Preparation

1. In a large skillet, heat the oil. Sauté the garlic until soft.
2. Add the shrimp. Season with paprika, salt, and pepper.
3. Cook until shrimp turn pink.
4. Serve. Garnish with chopped basil.

Nutrition Value

Calories: 278.3
Protein: 15.5g
Fat: 23.3g
Saturates: 1g
Carbs: 2.6g
Sugar: 0.5g
Fiber: 0.1g

21.Hot & Spicy Sweet Potato Salad

Prep time: 5 minutes. Cook time: 10 minutes. Servings: 2.

An ideal, spicy combination sure to temp any palette.

Ingredients

- 4 large sweet potatoes, diced into bite-size pieces
- 1 cup kidney beans
- 3 Tablespoons flavorless oil
- Pinch of salt and fresh ground pepper
- Red bell pepper, cored, seeded, diced

Dressing:

- ½ cup extra virgin olive oil
- ¼ cup red wine vinegar
- 2 teaspoons ground cumin
- ½ cup scallions, sliced
- 2 fresh chilies, minced
- Pinch of salt and pepper
- ¼ cup raisins (optional)
- 1 tablespoon grated orange zest
- ½ cup fresh mint leaves, minced

Preparation

Preheat oven to 400F

1. In a large bowl, add the bite-size sweet potatoes. Drizzle the 3 tablespoons of olive oil over them. Toss until evenly coated. Season with salt and pepper.
2. Spread the potatoes over a baking tray.
3. Place in the oven. Bake for 30 minutes, until fork tender. Turning half way through cooking.
4. As the potatoes bake, in a blender, combine the dressing ingredients.
5. Baste the potatoes at the halfway point with a couple tablespoons of the dressing.
6. Once potatoes cooked, pour them into a bowl. Add the dressing. Toss to evenly coat. Serve warm.

Nutrition Value

Calories: 333
Protein: 3.3g
Fat: 22.1g
Saturates: 1g
Carbs: 32.3g
Sugar: 0.5g
Fiber: 1g

22.Roasted Sweet Potatoes & Black Bean Burrito

Prep time: 5 minutes. Cook time: 55 minutes. Servings: 4.

There is no doubt this is delicious. The black beans! The jalapenos! The burrito! What a wonderful combination.

Ingredients

- 4 soft whole wheat tortilla wraps
- 4 sweet potatoes, diced
- 1 cup chopped tomatoes
- 3 Tbsp olive oil
- 2½ tsp ground cumin
- 1 red pepper, diced
- 1 jalapeno pepper, diced (seeds in or out, your choice)
- Pinch of salt and pepper
- ½ tsp cayenne pepper
- ½ can black beans, rinsed
- 1 cup frozen corn

Preparation

Preheat oven to 400 degrees

1. In a large bowl, add the chopped sweet potatoes. Drizzle olive oil over potatoes. Season with salt and pepper, and cumin.
2. Spread the potatoes in a single layer on a baking sheet.
3. Roast for 30 minutes.
4. After 30 minutes, add black beans, red pepper, tomatoes, corn. Drizzle more olive oil over the ingredients. Toss gently to evenly coat. Season with salt, pepper, and cumin.
5. Roast for an additional 20 minutes.
6. Wrap the soft tortillas in aluminum foil. Warm in oven 10 minutes.
7. Once everything is ready, place potatoe mixture in a large bowl. Place warm tortilla shell on a plate. Spoon potatoe mixture on wrap. Fold an end, roll the tortilla to form a burrito. Serve warm.

Nutrition Value

Calories: 123
Protein: 4.5g
Fat: 1.1g
Saturates: 2g
Carbs: 24.3g
Sugar: 2.2g
Fiber: 5.3g

23.Black & White Bean, Sweet Potato Soup

Prep time: 5 minutes. Cook time: 55 minutes. Servings: 4.

Black and white beans are whole grains considered very healthy and nutritious. A soup made with them is extra delicious.

Ingredients

- 1 Tbsp olive oil
- 1 onion, diced
- 1 garlic clove, minced
- 3 medium sweet potatoes
- 1 can navy beans, rinsed, drained
- 1 can black beans, rinsed, drained
- 1 small can diced tomatoes (don't rinse)
- 4 cups vegetable broth
- ¾ tsp ground cumin
- 2 Tbsp fresh lime juice
- ¾ tsp ground coriander
- Fresh ground pepper to taste

Preparation

1. In a large pot, drizzle in olive oil. Sauté onions and garlic 2 minutes.
2. Add the beans, tomatoes, potatoes to the pot. Cook for 5 minutes. Stirring occasionally.
3. Pour in the vegetable broth. Season pepper and cumin.
4. Simmer uncovered 25 minutes, until potatoes fork tender.
5. Add lemon juice towards the end. Serve hot.

Nutrition Value

Calories: 288
Protein: 12.3g
Fat: 3.9g
Saturates: 0.6g
Carbs: 50.7g
Sugar: 2.2g
Fiber: 11.3g

24.Collard Greens

Prep time: 40 minutes. Cook time: 25 minutes. Servings: 4.

Collard greens have held a vital place on the table for over a century. This recipe is yummy and easy to make.

Ingredients
- 2 Tbsp olive oil
- 3 garlic cloves, minced
- 1 small onion, thinly sliced
- ½ cup vegetable broth
- 2 Tbsp tomato puree
- 1 Tbsp balsamic vinegar
- ½ tsp salt
- 1 tsp sugar
- Bunch fresh of collard greens

Preparation
1. You will need a pressure cooker to make this recipe.
2. Collard greens must be thoroughly rinsed. Soak for 30 minutes, changing the water a few times during the process.
3. In pressure cooker, heat olive oil. Sauté onion and garlic 2 minutes.
4. Add vegetable broth, tomato puree, and vinegar. Stir until combined.
5. Remove thick stem from the greens. Tear into bite-size pieces.
6. Add to the pressure cooker. Cook for 20 minutes on high pressure.
7. Release pressure gently. Serve hot.

Nutrition Value
Calories: 49
Protein: 15.5g
Fat: 1.37g
Saturates: 1g
Carbs: 10.73g
Sugar: 0.5g
Fiber: 0.1g

25. Lentil Soup

Prep time: 5 minutes. Cook time: 15 minutes. Servings: 4.

Lentils coupled with vegetables are a perfect weekday dinner.

Ingredients

- 1 Tbsp olive oil
- 2 medium onions, finely chopped
- 2 garlic cloves, finely chopped
- 1 cup red lentils, rinsed
- 5 cups chicken broth
- 2 carrots, peeled, finely diced
- ½ tsp medium curry powder
- Dash of hot pepper paste
- Pinch of salt and pepper

Preparation

1. In a large saucepan, drizzle olive oil. Sauté onions, garlic 2 minutes.
2. Add the carrots. Sauté 2 minutes.
3. Add the lentils. Season with salt, pepper, curry powder, and hot pepper paste. Stir well. Add the vegetable broth.
4. Bring to boil. Cover and simmer 10 minutes.
5. Using a hand-held blender, pulse the ingredients to a thick soup consistency. Serve hot.

Nutrition Value

Calories: 186
Protein: 10.42g
Fat: 4.59g
Saturates: 0.593g
Carbs: 26.61g
Sugar: 2.38g
Fiber: 12.4g

26. Broccoli, Carrots, Peas, and Chard Stir Fry

Prep time: 5 minutes. Cook time: 15 minutes. Servings: 4.

Chard combined with broccoli, carrots, and peas creates this hearty stir fry.

Ingredients
- 1 medium head of broccoli, diced into florets
- 4 large carrots, diced
- 1 cup snow peas
- 5 leaves of chard, torn into small pieces
- 1 Tbsp butter
- Pinch of salt and pepper

Preparation
1. In a pot, steam the broccoli and carrots for 10 minutes.
2. Add snow peas. Steam another 5 minutes.
3. In a large frying pan, melt the butter without browning.
4. Add cooked vegetables. Add chard leaves. Stir.
5. Season with salt and pepper. Serve once leaves are wilted.

Nutrition Value
Calories: 80
Protein: 2g
Fat: 5g
Saturates: 1g
Carbs: 9g
Sugar: 5g
Fiber: 2g

27.Cauliflower Rice Stir Fry

Prep time: 5 minutes. Cook time: 15 minutes. Servings: 4.

With a mix of greens, this recipe stands out to be very nutritious.

Ingredients

Cauliflower rice

- 1 Tbsp coconut oil
- 1 white onion, diced
- 4 garlic cloves, minced
- Pinch coarse salt
- ¼ cup low sodium vegetable broth

Stir fry

- 1 Tbsp coconut oil
- 2 cups broccoli florets
- 1 large carrot, julienned
- ½ red bell pepper, diced
- 1 red onion, sliced
- 1 small red chili, sliced
- 1 Tbsp minced ginger
- Pinch of salt and pepper
- Juice from ½ lemon

Garnish

- 2 Tbsp pumpkin seeds, shelled
- 2 Tbsp fresh cilantro leaves, chopped

Preparation

1. Place the cauliflower florets in a food processor. Pulse until rice-like consistency is achieved.
2. In a large skillet, heat coconut oil. Sauté (diced) yellow onion and garlic 4 minutes.
3. Add cauliflower rice. Season with coarse salt. Stir in vegetable broth.
4. Simmer uncovered until broth is absorbed.
5. Place in a bowl. Cover.
6. Using the large skillet, heat 2 tablespoons coconut oil.
7. Add broccoli, carrots, bell pepper, red onion, and red chili. Season with salt, pepper, ginger. Stir well. Cook until vegetables fork tender.
8. Drizzle lemon juice over vegetables. Stir vegetables.
9. Spoon cauliflower rice into bowls. Spoon vegetables over cauliflower rice. Garnish with pumpkin seeds and cilantro leaves.

Nutrition Value

Calories: 57

Protein: 1g

Fat: 5g

Saturates: 1g

Carbs: 3g

Sugar: 1g

Fiber: 1g

28.Boiled Fowl with Rice

Prep time: 5 minutes. Cook time: 2-4 hours. Servings: 2.

For a substantial lunch, give this boiled fowl a chance.

Ingredients
- 1 cup basmati or jasmine rice
- A fowl suitable for boiling
- Pinch of salt and pepper
- 1 Tbsp butter

Preparation
1. Boil the fowl until tender, 2-4 hours.
2. Pull off cooked meat.
3. Cook rice according to package instructions.
4. Once cooked, season with butter, salt, and pepper.
5. Serve as a border around the fowl.

Nutrition Value
Calories: 254.1
Protein: 22.8g
Fat: 5g
Saturates: 1g
Carbs: 28.3g
Sugar: 0g
Fiber: 2.2g

29. Vegan Spaghetti with Anchovies

Prep time: 5 minutes. Cook time: 20 minutes. Servings: 2.

A hearty meal that will sustain you through the day.

Ingredients

- ½ package spaghetti
- 5 medium anchovies, diced
- 2 Tbsp olive oil
- 1 can diced tomatoes
- ¼ cup parmesan cheese, grated

Preparation

1. Place anchovies in a colander. Steam in boiling water to loosen skin. Skin and de-bone completely. Dice anchovies.
2. In large sauce pan, pour in can of tomatoes. Simmer 5 minutes. Add the anchovies. Stir. Turn heat off, leave pot on element.
3. Cook spaghetti according to package instructions; el dante.
4. Place spaghetti in large serving dish. Pour sauce over the spaghetti.
5. Toss the sauce and pasta. Top with grated cheese.

Nutrition Value

Calories: 411
Protein: 9.6g
Fat: 19g
Saturates: 1g
Carbs: 51g
Sugar: 1.7g
Fiber: 1.9g

Prep time: 15 minutes. Cook time: 30 minutes. Servings: 4.

This Indian-spiced chard makes a perfect main dish.

Ingredients

- 1 tsp cumin powder
- 1 onion, diced
- 3 garlic cloves, minced
- 1 tomato, chopped
- 1 tsp masala
- ¼ cup water
- 3 Tbsp olive oil
- 17 leaves rainbow chard
- 1 Tbsp minced ginger
- 1 tsp turmeric
- ½ tsp red chili flakes
- 1 tsp kosher salt
- 1 block cubed extra firm tofu
- ¼ cup fresh cilantro, rough chopped
- ¼ cup roasted cashews

Preparation

1. Pull chard off the stalks, rip into pieces. Rinse well.
2. In a large pan, heat olive oil. Sauté garlic, onions, and ginger 3 minutes.
3. Add cleaned chard. Cook 2 minutes.
4. Add masala, red chili flakes, salt, and turmeric. Cook 5 minutes.
5. Add diced tomato. Cook until softened. Add water.
6. Reduce heat. Add tofu.
7. Cook on low heat 20 minutes, until tofu is tender.
8. Serve in bowls. Garnish with cilantro leaves and cashews.

Nutrition Value

Calories: 57
Protein: 1g
Fat: 5g
Saturates: 1g
Carbs: 3g
Sugar: 1g
Fiber: 1g

31.Polenta & Beans Mix

Prep time: 5 minutes. Cook time: 35 minutes. Servings: 4.

Polenta and beans make a great, easy meal.

Ingredients

Beans

- 2 Tbsp extra virgin olive oil
- 1 Tbsp fresh flat leaf parsley, finely chopped
- 2 garlic cloves, minced
- 1 can diced tomatoes
- 1 tsp chopped fresh sage
- 1 can cannellini beans, rinsed, drained
- ¼ tsp each - salt and fresh ground pepper

Polenta

- 4 cups water
- ¼ tsp salt
- 1 cup coarse yellow dry polenta

Garnish:

Fresh parsley

Preparation

1. In a large saucepan over medium heat, heat olive oil. Add garlic and parsley. Cook 60 seconds.
2. Add tomatoes, beans, and sage. Stir. Cook until liquid evaporates, approximately 10 minutes.
3. As tomatoes and beans cook, in a separate pot, boil water with salt.
4. Add the polenta. Cover and cook 6 minutes, uncover, stir with a fork. Cover. Cook 2 minutes. Uncover, fluff with fork.
5. Serve the polenta in bowls. Top with bean mixture. Garnish with fresh parsley.

Nutrition Value

Calories: 284
Protein: 11.1g
Fat: 1.8g
Saturates: 0.2g
Carbs: 56.7g
Sugar: 8.4g
Fiber: 10.4g

32.Vegan Split Pea & Sweet Potato Soup

Prep time: 15 minutes. Cook time: 1 hour 20 minutes. Servings: 4.

The soup is easy to make and nutritious.

Ingredients
- 2 cups split yellow peas
- 1 Tbsp flavorless oil
- 1 medium yellow onion, chopped
- 4 cups vegetable broth
- 2 medium sweet potatoes, peeled, diced into ½ inch pieces
- 7 whole green cardamom pods
- ¼ tsp cayenne pepper
- ½ tsp ground cumin
- 1 tsp masala
- Dash of lemon juice
- ⅛ tsp fine sea salt
- ¼ cup coconut milk
- Pinch of fresh ground black pepper

Preparation
1. Soak peas overnight. Drain as you rinse them.
2. In a large saucepan, heat the oil. Sauté onion for 2 minutes.
3. Add the diced potato, beans, and cardamom pods. Stir in the vegetable broth.
4. Cover and simmer for 30 minutes.
5. In a small skillet, heat the ghee. Add the masala, cayenne pepper, and cumin. Heat for 5 minutes.
6. Add to the beans and potatoes. Stir in coconut milk.
7. Remove the cardamom pods. Heat the soup until it thickens.

Nutrition Value
Calories: 254
Protein: 2.1g
Fat: 3.9g
Saturates: 0.5g
Carbs: 40.2g
Sugar: 7.1g
Fiber: 15.5g

*33.*Taco Salad In A Mason jar

(Prep time: 10 minutes\ Cook time: 20 minutes| 2 servings)

While usually we use mason jars to store pickles, in this recipe we are going to be using our Mason Jar to store a finely prepared Taco Salad!

Ingredients:

- 2 -3 Tablespoons olive oil
- 8 ounce chicken breast, cut into bite sized pieces
- 2 carrots, sliced
- 1 large red bell pepper, sliced
- ½ onion, roughly chopped
- 2 garlic cloves, minced
- 2 teaspoons of cumin seed
- 1 large avocado, diced
- Juice from 1 lime
- 1 cup of salsa
- 2 cups Roma tomatoes, chopped
- ½ cucumber, chopped
- ½ cup cilantro, roughly chopped
- ½ cup fresh spinach, roughly chopped
- 2 quart wide-mouth mason jars
- Pinch of salt and pepper

Preparation:

1) In a large skillet, pour in 1 tablespoon olive oil, heat it over medium.
2) Add the garlic and onion. Sauté until translucent.
3) Toss in the chicken breast, cook until golden brown.
4) Drizzle oil into pan with chicken. Add the carrots. Cook for 3 minutes.
5) Reduce heat to low, add bell pepper.
6) In a separate pan, over medium /high heat toast the cumin seeds for 2 minutes. Gently transfer them from there to a cutting board. Crush them gently. Add the seeds to the pan of chicken and vegetables.
7) Dice the avocado. Place in food processor. Pour in the lime juice. Pulse until smooth.
8) Then take your mason jar and pour ½ cup of salsa in the bottom. Pour in avocado mixture next.
9) Add the chicken and vegetables next. Add a layer of tomatoes, cucumbers, cilantro, and spinach leaves. When ready to eat, toss with your favorite paleo-friendly dressing.

Nutrition Values

- Calories: 177
- Fat: 9.1g
- Carbohydrates: 9.8g
- Protein: 16g
- Dietary Fiber: 4.7g

34.Lettuce Tacos with Chipotle Chicken

(Prep time: 20 minutes\ Cook time: 30 minutes| 4 servings)

If you are in the mood for chicken and something crunchy, this recipe will satisfy both cravings. The Chipotle chicken is perfect with your lettuce Tacos.

Ingredients:

- 2 large chicken breasts, sliced
- 2 – 3 Tablespoons of olive oil
- 1 red onion, finely sliced
- 2 garlic cloves, minced
- 1 small tin of diced tomatoes
- 1 teaspoon of finely chopped chipotle
- ½ teaspoon of cumin
- Pinch of brown sugar
- 8 – 10 leaves Large lettuce
- Fresh coriander leaves
- Sliced up pickled jalapeno chilies
- Slices of guacamole
- 1 tomato, sliced
- Lime wedges

Preparation:

1) In a large frying pan, drizzle oil over bottom of pan. Sauté the sliced onion and garlic until translucent.
2) Add the chicken. Cook until golden brown. Set aside.
3) Add tomatoes, brown sugar, cumin, chipotle to pan. Simmer 10 minutes, until tomato fork tender and a sauce starts to form.
4) Return chicken to the pan. Stir until chicken evenly coated. Simmer for 5 minutes.
5) Assemble rest of ingredients in bowls to make tacos.
6) Place a lettuce leaf on a plate. Top with chicken. Option to add other toppings: pickled jalapeno, guacamole, fresh tomato slice. Drizzle lime juice over ingredients.

Nutrition Values

- Calories: 332
- Fat: 15.7g
- Carbohydrates: 13.9g
- Protein: 34.3g
- Dietary Fiber: 2.1g

35.Spicy Picadillo Lettuce Wrap

(Prep time: 10 minutes\ Cook time: 25 minutes| 6 servings)

Yet another recipe involving Lettuce Wrap, but this time a little bit more over the top with finely crafted Paleo suitable Lettuce Tacos!

Ingredients:

For the Picadillo

- 1 pound of grass fed ground beef
- 2 Tablespoons of coconut oil
- 1 onion, diced
- 1 garlic clove, minced
- ½ teaspoon of salt
- 1 teaspoon fresh ground black pepper
- 1 teaspoon of ground cumin
- ½ teaspoon of ground cinnamon
- 1 x 14 ounce can whole tomatoes
- ¼ cup of currants
- 2 Tablespoons of green olives
- 2 Tablespoons of drained capers
- 2 Tablespoons of olive brine

For the Pico De Gallo

- ½ cup of minced red onion
- ⅔ cup of diced tomatoes
- 2 Tablespoons of minced cilantro
- 2 teaspoons of fresh lime juice
- Pinch of salt, pepper

Serving

- Large leaf lettuce
- Cooked brown rice
- Chopped cilantro

Preparation:

1) In a large frying pan, drizzle oil over bottom. Sauté onion and garlic for 1 minute. Add the ground beef. Break into small pieces. Cook until no longer pink in middle.
2) Add the bell pepper. Cook until fork tender.
3) In a separate pot, heat the canned tomatoes, currants, diced olives, olive brine, and capers. Add the cooked beef. Stir until combined. Bring to a boil, cook for 5 minutes.
4) Reduce temperature to simmer 10-20 minutes.
5) On the side, prepare the ingredients listed for pico de Gallo.
6) On a plate, place a large leaf of lettuce. Spoon on cooked beef, cooked rice. Garnish with fresh cilantro. Top with pico de Gallo.

Nutrition Values

- Calories: 178
- Fat: 7.8g
- Carbohydrates: 7.8g
- Protein: 20.5g
- Dietary Fiber: 1.5g

36.California Turkey, Bacon Lettuce Wrap with Basil Mayo

(Prep time: 10 minutes\ Cook time: nil| 2 servings)

Mixing up a fine lettuce wrap with the juicy goodness of bacon and basil mayo for an added oomph factor.

Ingredients:

For the Wrap

- 1 head of iceberg lettuce
- 4 slices of gluten-free deli turkey
- 3 slices of gluten-free bacon, cooked
- 1 avocado, thinly sliced
- 1 Roma tomato, thinly sliced

Serving

- ½ cup of gluten-free mayonnaise
- 6 large basil leaves, torn
- 1 teaspoon lemon juice
- 1 garlic clove, chopped
- Pinch of salt and pepper

Preparation:

1) In a food processor, combine the ingredients for basil mayo. Pulse until smooth consistency.
2) Place a large leaf of lettuce on a plate. Layer a slice of turkey, slice of bacon, slice of tomato, then a slice of avocado. Spread mayo over ingredients. Season with salt and pepper.
3) Tuck the ends in, roll the lettuce leaf over your filling, creating a burrito.
4) Slice in half. Serve chilled.

Nutrition Values

- Calories: 150
- Fat: 13.5g
- Carbohydrates: 17.5g
- Protein: 6.1g
- Dietary Fiber: 4g

(Prep time: 10 minutes\ Cook time: 10 minutes| 1 servings)

A proper meal cannot be complete without having a few pieces of steak with it, right? This recipe gives you that and more in the form of steak wrapped around in fresh wrap.

Ingredients:

- ½ pound of fajita seasoned steak strips (cut in ½ inch strips)
- 1 small onion, sliced
- 2 garlic cloves, diced
- 1 small bell pepper, diced
- 2 Tablespoons of siracha sauce
- 2 teaspoons of coconut aminos
- Sesame seed oil
- Green onions for garnish
- A handful of pea shoots
- 2 – 4 Large leaves of romaine lettuce

Preparation:

1) Drizzle oil along bottom of a large frying pan. Add the onion and garlic. Sauté on medium for 2 minutes until translucent.
2) Add the sliced fajita steak. Cook 2 minutes per side.
3) Add the bell pepper. Cook until fork tender.
4) Drizzle in more sesame seed oil. Add the pea shoots, coconut aminos, and Sirach sauce. Stir well.
5) Once the meat has absorbed the sauce, turn off the heat.
6) Spoon the mixture into lettuce leaves. Garnish with diced green onions. Serve hot.

Nutrition Values

- Calories: 268
- Fat: 13.5g
- Carbohydrates: 17.9g
- Protein: 1.9g
- Dietary Fiber: 19.3g

38. Cajun Shrimp Noodle Bowl

(Prep time: 5 minutes\ Cook time: 15 minutes| 2 servings)

Coming straight from the Mexican tables, this shrimp cajun delight might be a bit spicy, but definitely worth the effort! Easily made to satisfy your shrimp lust!

Ingredients:

For the Dish

- 3 garlic cloves, crushed
- 3 Tablespoons of grass fed butter
- 20 jumbo shrimp, deveined, tail off

For the Cajun Seasoning

- 1 teaspoon of paprika
- Dash of cayenne pepper
- ½ teaspoon of Himalayan Sea Salt
- Dash of red pepper flakes
- 1 teaspoon of garlic granules
- 1 teaspoon of onion powder

For Others

- 1 large zucchini, spiralized
- 1 red pepper, sliced
- 1 onion, thinly sliced
- 1 Tablespoon of grass fed butter

Preparation:

1) Spiralize the Zucchini.
2) In a large bowl, add the cajun seasoning. Add the shrimp. Toss until evenly coated with seasoning.
3) Heat a large frying pan on medium. Melt the butter. Add the garlic, onion, and red pepper. Sauté for 2 minutes.
4) Add the shrimp. Cook until shrimp turns pink.
5) In a separate frying pan, heat up the butter. Lightly sauté the Zucchini noodles for approximately 3 minutes – el dante.
6) Place the Zucchini noodles in a bowl. Top with garlic Cajun shrimp and vegetable mixture

Nutrition Values

- Calories: 92
- Fat: 7.6g
- Carbohydrates: 2.2g
- Protein: 4.6g
- Dietary Fiber: 0.8g

39.Egg Roll In A Bowl
(Prep time: 10 minutes\ Cook time: 10 minutes| 2 servings)

Looking for a quick fix to your Paleo Hunger? Serve up a plate of Paleo egg roll for a quick lunch to maintain your diet and get back to your busy life.

Ingredients:

- 1 small head of a cabbage, chopped into slices
- 1 skinless, boneless chicken breast, diced in bite-size pieces
- 2 large carrots
- 1 Tablespoon of unflavored coconut oil
- ⅓ cup of coconut aminos
- 1 Tablespoon of sesame seed oil
- 2 garlic cloves, minced
- 4 green onions, diced

Preparation:

1) In a large frying pan, heat up the coconut oil over medium-high heat.
2) Add the garlic. Sauté for 1 minute. Add the chicken. Cook until no longer pink in middle – depending on thickness, anywhere from 5 – 7 minutes.
3) Toss in the cabbage and carrots. Sauté until vegetables are fork tender. (You don't want them too soft. A bit of a crunch is good.)
4) Add the coconut aminos. Stir until the ingredients are coated. Simmer for a minute or two until sauce absorbed.
5) Serve into bowls. Garnish with diced green onions.

Nutrition Values

Calories: 463 Fat: 18.5g Carbohydrates: 27.8g Protein: 49.8g Dietary Fiber: 9.3g

40.Anti-Pasto Salad

(Prep time: 5 minutes\ Cook time: nil| 4 servings)

A hearty salad to fill any craving.

Ingredients:

- 1 large romaine lettuce, chopped into chunks
- ½ cup prosciutto, chopped into chunks
- ½ cup salami, chopped into cubes
- ½ cup of artichoke, chopped into chunks
- ½ cup black olives, whole
- ½ cup of hot or sweet peppers, whole
- Italian dressing as required

Preparation:

1) Add all the ingredients to a large bowl.
2) Drizzle in dressing. Toss until evenly coated.
3) Serve in bowls.

Nutrition Values

Calories: 240 Fat: 13g Carbohydrates: 19g Protein: 2g Dietary Fiber: 0g

CHAPTER 4: MEAL PREP FOR DINNER

41.Rabbit with Mustard

Prep time: 15 minutes. Cook time: 75 minutes. Servings: 4.

Imagine how impressed your guests would be if you served this for dinner. Or how about your family.

Ingredients (for one rabbit):

- 1 whole rabbit
- ½ cup Dijon mustard
- 3 Tbsp olive oil
- 2 garlic cloves, minced
- 5 shallots, diced
- 3 bay leaves
- 1 sprig of thyme
- ¼ tsp fresh parsley, chopped
- 1 bottle of dry white wine
- Pinch of salt, pepper
- 1 carrot, diced
- 1 cup cooking cream

Preparation

1. Dice the rabbit into sections. Lightly brush with mustard.
2. In a large skillet, heat 2 tablespoons of the olive oil. Sear the rabbit on both sides.
3. In a large saucepan, heat up 1 tablespoon of the oil. Sauté the garlic, shallots, carrot, thyme for 3 minutes. Pour in the wine. Stir.
4. Add the rabbit to the wine mixture. Add the bay leaves.
5. Cover and simmer on medium for 60 minutes.
6. After 60 minutes, add the cream to the pot. Turn the heat up, stir as the sauce thickens.
7. When cooked, place the rabbit pieces in a serving bowl. Serve hot.

Nutrition Value

Calories: 523

Protein: 99g

Fat: 10g

Saturates: 3g

Carbs: 1 g

Sugar: 0g

Fiber: 3.1g

42. Vegan Tofu Vegetable Stir Fry

Prep time: 15 minutes. Cook time: 20 minutes. Servings: 4.

Vegetables and tofu. You need to try this!

Ingredients
- 2 cups tofu, cubed
- 2 Tbsp olive oil
- 3 green onions, sliced
- ½ cup beansprouts
- ½ cup cherry tomatoes
- 1 red bell pepper, sliced
- 1 orange bell pepper, sliced
- 1 yellow bell pepper, sliced
- 1 tsp diced ginger
- Fresh ground pepper
- ¼ cup roasted cashews

Preparation
1. Cut the tofu into cubes. Marinate with 1 tablespoon of salt.
2. Heat oil in wok. Add the vegetables and ginger. Cook for 10 minutes, while stirring. Add the tofu cubes and heat 5 minutes.
3. Serve in bowls. Garnish with cashews.

Nutrition Value
Calories: 364
Protein: 35g
Fat: 3.9g
Saturates: 0.5g
Carbs: 20g
Sugar: 7.1g
Fiber: 7.5g

43.Paleo Chickpeas with Cumin

Prep time: 15 minutes. Cook time: 10 minutes. Servings: 4.

Turn chickpeas into lunch!

Ingredients
- Juice from 1 lemon
- 1 garlic clove, minced
- 1 bunch flat leaf parsley, rough chopped
- 2 cups chickpeas (if using canned, rinse under cold water)
- ¼ cup kidney beans
- 2 potatoes, peeled, diced
- 1 carrot, peeled, diced
- 3 Tbsp olive oil
- 1 Tbsp ground cumin
- 1 Tbsp paprika
- Pinch of salt and pepper

Preparation
1. In a large saucepan, heat the oil. Sauté garlic 1 minute.
2. Add the chickpeas, kidney beans, potatoe, and carrot. Cook 10 minutes, until potato fork tender.
3. In a bowl, combine fresh squeezed lemon juice, parsley, paprika, cumin, pepper. Stir. Pour over the chickpeas mixture. Stir to coat evenly.
4. Serve in bowls. Garnish with fresh parsley.

Nutrition Value
Calories: 268
Protein: 12.5g
Fat: 4.2g
Saturates: 0.5g
Carbs: 20g
Sugar: 7.1g
Fiber: 14.5g

44.Grilled Swordfish with Herbs

Prep time: 15 minutes. Cook time: 20 minutes. Servings: 4.

Grilled sword fish with herbs makes a perfect combination and meal.

Ingredients
- 12oz swordfish
- 1 sprig of thyme
- Pinch of salt and fresh ground pepper
- 1 Tbsp olive oil
- Juice from ½ lemon
- Orange and lemon wedges

Preparation
1. Brush swordfish with olive oil. Season with lemon juice, salt, pepper.
2. In a large skillet, fry the fish 3 minutes per side. Add thyme to pan.
3. Cover the skillet. Let the fish rest for 5 minutes.
4. Serve with lemon and orange wedges.

Nutrition Value
Calories: 165
Protein: 21.8g
Fat: 6.8g
Saturates: 1.5g
Carbs: 2.5g
Sugar: 7.1g
Fiber: 0.2g

45.Fish Fillets with Sesame

Prep time: 15 minutes. Cook time: 20 minutes. Servings: 4.

Easy to make, delicious, and nutritious: basically a recipe of clean eating for dummies.

Ingredients

- Sesame oil or vegetable oil
- 4 Haddock fillets
- Grated orange zest
- Pinch of salt and pepper
- ¾ cup sesame seeds
- 1 package fresh spinach, rough chopped
- 2 Tbsp butter

Preparation

Preheat broiler to 450F

1. In a bowl, using a whisk, combine oil, orange zest, salt, and pepper. Brush mixture on each side of fish fillets.
2. Place the sesame seeds on a plate. Rotate the fish in the sesame seeds.
3. Place fish fillets on a baking tray. Cook under preheated broiler, 6 inches away from element, 5 minutes per side.
4. In a skillet, heat the butter. Add the spinach leaves. Season with salt and pepper. Stir until wilted.
5. Divide spinach between 4 plates. Serve the fish on top.

Nutrition Value

Calories: 276
Protein: 42.3g
Fat: 7.8g
Saturates: 1.5g
Carbs: 7.5g
Sugar: 7.1g
Fiber: 2.7g

46.Chickpea Soup

Prep time: 15 minutes. Cook time: 25 minutes. Servings: 4.

Creamy coconut curried soup is a hearty favorite for many people.

Ingredients

- 3 Tbsp olive oil
- 1 yellow onion, diced
- 2 cups chickpeas, cooked
- 2 potatoes, peeled, diced
- 2 cups vegetable broth
- 2 Tbsp curry paste
- 1 cup coconut milk
- 1 bunch kale
- Optional: Juice from 1 lime

Instruction

1. In a large saucepan, heat the oil. Sauté onion 4 minutes.
2. Add chickpeas, diced potatoes.
3. Stir in vegetable broth, curry paste. Simmer 10 minutes.
4. Stir in coconut milk. Add kale. Simmer 10 minutes.
5. Serve in bowls. Optional: squeeze in lime juice.

Nutrition Value

Calories: 359
Protein: 25.3g
Fat: 12.1g
Saturates: 1g
Carbs: 22.3g
Sugar: 0.5g
Fiber: 1g

47.Fresh Salmon with Vegetables

Prep time: 15 minutes. Cook time: 30 minutes. Servings 4.

Salmon. It's simply delicious and perfect clean eating.

Ingredients

- 4 salmon fillets (15 oz each)
- Juice from 1 lemon
- 2 tomatoes, diced
- 1 onion, diced
- 1 chili green diced
- 2 garlic cloves, minced
- 1 Tbsp flavorless oil
- Pinch of salt and pepper

Preparation

Preheat oven to 350F

1. Place salmon fillets in a bowl. Season with lemon, salt, and pepper.
2. In another bowl, combine the tomatoes, onion, chili, garlic. Drizzle oil over ingredients. Season with salt and pepper. Stir.
3. Place the fish in a single layer in a glass baking dish. Pour the tomato mixture over the fish.
4. Bake 30 minutes, until fish is flaky.

Nutrition Value

Calories: 366.7
Protein: 45.2g
Fat: 15g
Saturates: 2.6g
Carbs: 11.3g
Sugar: 3.2g
Fiber: 1.9g

48.Quinoa with Vegetables

Prep time: 15 minutes. Cook time: 30 minutes. Servings: 2.

Light and citrusy, perfect new way to enjoy quinoa.

Ingredients

- ¼ cup quinoa
- 1 large tomato, diced
- 1 red pepper, diced
- ¼ cup niblets corn
- 1 small onion, diced
- 2 avocados, diced
- Bunch of fresh coriander
- Juice from 2 limes
- 2 Tbsp olive oil
- Salt and pepper

Preparation

1. Rinse the quinoa.
2. Cook the quinoa in 2 times its volume, in water.
3. Bring to a boil. Reduce heat and cook for 20 minutes. Let it cool.
4. Cut vegetables into small cubes.
5. Thin out and chop the coriander.
6. Prepare vinaigrette of olive oil and lemon juice. Season the vegetables.
7. Mix the vegetables with the quinoa. Stir. Serve.

Nutrition Value

Calories: 202
Protein: 7.4g
Fat: 3g
Saturates: 1.3g
Carbs: 37.5g
Sugar: 3.5g
Fiber: 7.1g

49. Grilled Salmon with Peppers

Prep time: 15 minutes. Cook time: 30 minutes. Servings: 4.

The simplest and delicious way to eat salmon.

Ingredients

- 21 oz. fillet salmon without skin
- 1 red bell pepper, sliced
- 1 green bell pepper, sliced
- 1 yellow bell pepper, sliced
- 1 clove garlic, minced
- Few sprigs of mint
- Juice from 1 lemon
- 6 Tbsp olive oil
- Pinch of salt and pepper

Preparation

1. Spread a thin layer of oil over the salmon fillet. Season with salt and pepper. Cook the salmon in a pan, or under the broiler.
2. In a skillet, heat some olive oil. Sauté garlic 2 minutes. Add sliced bell peppers to skillet. Season with salt and pepper. Cook until tender.
3. Once the fish is cooked, take it out of the oven, drizzle lemon juice over the fillet. Let it rest 2 minutes.
4. Transfer cooked peppers to serving dish. Place salmon fillet over top. Garnish with fresh mint leaves.

Nutrition Value

Calories: 199
Protein: 14.6g
Fat: 2.5g
Saturates: 2.1g
Carbs: 11.9g
Sugar: 2.8g
Fiber: 4g

50.Skillet Chicken Thighs With Butternut Squash

(Prep time: 15 minutes\ Cook time: 30 minutes| 4-6 servings)

Butternut are pretty famous for their nice flavor. If you have a skillet lying around this dish can be whipped up in no time.

Ingredients:

- ½ pound of Nitrate free bacon
- 6 boneless, skinless chicken thighs
- 2 - 3 cups of butternut squash, cubed
- Extra virgin olive oil/ coconut oil for frying
- Fresh sage, finely chopped
- Salt and pepper

Preparation:

Preheat oven to 425F
1) In a large skillet over medium-high heat, fry bacon until crispy.
2) Set bacon aside. Crumble when cooled.
3) In same skillet, using the bacon grease, sauté butternut squash for a few minutes, until el dante. Season with salt and pepper.
4) Once the squash is el dante, remove from skillet.
5) Add coconut oil to skillet (if bacon grease is low).
6) Add the chicken thighs; season with salt and pepper.
7) Cook for 10 minutes until no longer pink in middle.
8) Flip them over. Return butternut squash to skillet.
9) Place skillet in preheated oven. Bake for 12 - 15 minutes, until butternut squash is fork tender.
10) Remove skillet from oven. Top with crumbled bacon and sage. Serve hot.

Nutrition Values

- Calories: 323
- Fat: 19g
- Carbohydrates: 15g
- Protein: 12g
- Dietary Fiber: 5.2g

51.Sweet Potato Turkey Casserole W/Eggplant and Tomato

(Prep time: 15 minutes\ Cook time: 60 minutes| 6 servings)

People don't usually consider Eggplant to be a delicious ingredient. But mix it up with sweet potato and turkey, and you have one heck of a hearty meal with a tangy kick from the tomato.

Ingredients:

For the Casserole

- 1 pound of extra lean ground turkey
- 1 medium sweet potato, peeled, diced into small pieces
- 1 medium eggplant, sliced in ½ inch pieces
- 1 Tablespoon extra-virgin olive oil
- ½ onion, chopped
- 1 garlic clove, minced
- 1 x 15 ounce can diced tomatoes
- 1 x 8 ounce can tomato paste
- Salt and pepper to taste
- ¼ teaspoon of chili powder
- ¼ teaspoon of cumin
- ⅛ teaspoon of oregano
- ⅛ teaspoon of ground cardamom
- ½ teaspoon of tarragon flakes

For the Sauce

- 1½ Tablespoons extra-virgin olive oil
- 1 cup of unsweetened almond milk
- 1 Tablespoon of almond flour
- 1 Tablespoon of coconut flour

Preparation:

Preheat oven to 350F

1) Spray an 8x8 baking/casserole dish with non-stick cooking spray.
2) Heat a large pan over medium heat. Drizzle in olive oil. Sauté onion and garlic for 2 minutes.
3) Add the turkey. Using a wooden spoon, break up the turkey and brown the meat until no longer pink. Add the sweet potatoes.
4) Stir in tomatoes and tomato paste until ingredients evenly coated.
5) Continue cooking until sweet potato pieces are el dante.
6) In a bowl, combine chili powder, cumin, oregano, cardamom, tarragon, salt and pepper. Add eggplant. Stir until eggplant coated.
7) Place eggplant in a single layer along bottom of baking dish.
8) Top with turkey and sweet potato mix. Bake for 15 minutes.
9) In a small pot, heat up the olive oil. Add the coconut flour and almond flour. Stir for 1 – 2 minutes to cook the flour. Whisk in the almond milk slowly. Stir until fully incorporated. Bring to a boil, stirring constantly. Mixture will thicken and reduce.
10) Pull the baking dish out of oven. Pour mixture over ingredients. Return to oven. Bake another 30 minutes, until top is golden brown.
11) Remove from oven. Slice into 6 servings. Garnish with fresh tarragon.

Nutrition Values

Calories: 278 Fat: 2.6g Carbohydrates: 15g Protein: 28.5g Dietary Fiber: 28.5g

52.Paleo Pizza Soup
(Prep time: 5 minutes\ Cook time: 30 minutes| 6 servings)

Pizza as a soup? Surprise your guests with this unique concoction that combines the flavors of pizza and delights of your favorite soup.

Ingredients:

- 1 cup chicken sausage, sliced
- ½ cup uncured pepperoni
- 1 x 25 ounce jar marinara sauce
- 1 x 14.5 ounce can fire roasted tomatoes
- ¼ cup vegetable or beef broth, no salt added
- 1 Tablespoon any flavorless oil
- 1 onion, diced
- 2 garlic cloves, minced
- ½ cup mushrooms, sliced
- 1 x 3 ounce can sliced black olives
- 1 Tablespoon of dried oregano
- 1 teaspoon of garlic powder
- Pinch of salt and pepper

Preparation:

1) In a large saucepan, heat up the oil. Sauté the onion and garlic for 2 minutes, until translucent.
2) Add sausage, peperoni, mushrooms, olives, and tomatoes to pot. Stir well. Brown until sausage and peperoni cooked through.
3) Add marinara sauce and vegetable/or beef broth. Stir in oregano, garlic powder, salt and pepper.
4) Simmer on low-medium heat approximately 30 minutes, until mushrooms are tender.
5) Serve hot

Nutrition Values

- Calories: 90
- Fat: 2g
- Carbohydrates: 17g
- Protein: 3g
- Dietary Fiber: 3g

53.Spicy Pumpkin Chili

(Prep time: 10 minutes\ Cook time: 15 minutes| 5 servings)

This recipe will give you the perfect blend of pumpkin with just the right amount of spicy goodness to satisfy the dragon in you.

Ingredients:

- 1 Tablespoon flavorless oil
- 2 yellow onions, chopped
- 8 garlic cloves, chopped
- 1 pound of lean ground turkey
- 2 x 15 ounce cans fire roasted tomatoes
- 2 cups of pumpkin puree
- 1 cup of chicken broth
- 2 Tablespoons of honey
- 4 teaspoons of chili spice
- 1 teaspoon of ground cinnamon
- 1 teaspoon of sea salt

Preparation:

1) In a large pot, heat the oil. Sauté onion and garlic for 2-4 minutes.
2) Add ground turkey. Using a wooden spoon, break up into small pieces. Cook until no longer pink.
3) Add the tomatoes and pumpkin puree to pot. Stir well.
4) Stir in the honey, chili spice, cinnamon, sea salt, and chicken broth. Simmer 15 minutes without a lid.
5) Serve in bowls.

Nutrition Values

- Calories: 312
- Fat: 16.2g
- Carbohydrates: 13.5g
- Protein: 27.4g
- Dietary Fiber: 27.4g

54.Creamy Basil And Tomato Chicken

(Prep time: 10 minutes\ Cook time: 20 minutes| 4 servings)

This recipe will give you the perfect meal if you are looking for something a little bit tangy, but has the benefits of green vegetables and protein punch of chicken.

Ingredients:

- 1 pound boneless, skinless chicken breast, diced
- ½ yellow onion
- 1 teaspoon of coconut oil
- 3 garlic cloves
- 2 Tablespoons of sunflower seeds
- 1 Tablespoon of nutritional yeast
- 1 package of fresh basil
- 1 Tablespoon of avocado oil
- Salt and pepper to taste
- ½ cup of coconut milk
- ½ teaspoon of arrowroot powder
- ⅓ cup of cold water
- 1 cup cherry tomatoes, sliced

Preparation:

1) In a large skillet, heat up the coconut oil. Add the onion and garlic. Cook for 2 minutes, until translucent.
2) Add the chicken. Cook for 12 minutes, flipping at the halfway point.
3) In the meantime, take a plate and toss in the garlic in a food processor bowl to finely mince it using the processor
4) Pour in the sunflower seeds. Pulse again, until sand-like consistency.
5) Add the nutritional yeast, salt, and pepper. Pulse until fully minced.
6) In a medium bowl, whisk the arrowroot powder with a few drops of water, to create a paste.
7) Pour in the coconut milk. Whisk until combined.
8) Pour sauce into the skillet. Stir well. Bring to a simmer.
9) Add in the sliced cherry tomatoes. Simmer 1-2 minutes. Serve hot.

Nutrition Values

- Calories: 408
- Fat: 31g
- Carbohydrates: 9g
- Protein: 23g
- Dietary Fiber: 3g

55.Amazing Ground Turkey and Spinach Stuffed Mushroom

(Prep time: 10 minutes\ Cook time: 15 minutes| 2 servings)

Ground turkey stuffed in portobello mushrooms creates something truly delicious that is both meaty and healthy with the power of Popeye's Spinach.

Ingredients:

- 2 teaspoons of coconut oil
- 6 large Portobello mushrooms, caps cleared and gills removed.
- 1 small onion, diced
- ½ pound of lean ground turkey
- Handful of baby spinach leaves
- 6-8 grape tomatoes, sliced
- Salt and pepper to taste

Preparation:

1) In a large skillet, heat up 1 teaspoon of coconut oil. Heat the mushroom caps 2 minutes per side, until soft. Set aside.
2) Drizzle more oil in skillet. Sauté onion on medium heat for 2 minutes.
3) In the same skillet, add the ground turkey to the pan, break it up into small pieces. Cook until no longer pink. Season with salt and pepper.
4) Once cooked, remove the meat. Place tomato slices and spinach in the skillet. Heat until tomatoes soft and spinach wilted. Return meat to the pan. Stir until combined.
5) Using a spoon, scoop filling into the mushroom caps. Serve hot.

Nutrition Values

- Calories: 220
- Fat: 46g
- Carbohydrates: 14g
- Protein: 25g
- Dietary Fiber: 5g

56.Shepherd's Pie with Cauliflower Topping
(Prep time: 30 minutes\ Cook time: 30 minutes| 4-6 servings)

Shepherd's pie with cauliflower? Now, that's a twist!

Ingredients:

- 1 head of cauliflower, chopped into florets
- 4 Tablespoons of ghee
- 1 small onion, diced
- 2 stalks of celery, diced
- 2 garlic cloves, minced
- 1 pound of lean ground beef
- ¼ - 1/2 cup of homemade beef broth
- 1 Tablespoon of homemade ketchup
- 2 Tablespoons of fresh parsley, rough chopped
- Salt and pepper to taste
- ½ - ¾ cup shredded cheddar cheese

Preparation:

Preheat oven to 400
1) Grease an 8-inch square casserole/baking dish.
2) In a large pot, steam the cauliflower until tender.
3) In a large skillet, heat up 1 tablespoon of ghee.
4) Add the onion, garlic, celery, garlic, and carrot to the skillet. Cook for 5 minutes, until vegetables are tender.
5) Add the ground beef. Brown until no longer pink. Add beef broth a bit at a time, so the meat remains wet but not saturated.
6) Add the ketchup. Season with salt and pepper. Simmer as you prepare the cauliflower.
7) Place the cauliflower in a blender. Pulse until it is smooth. Pour in 1 tablespoon of ghee. Pulse again. Season with salt and pepper. Add parsley. Stir well.
8) Assembling: Spread a layer of meat mixture along bottom of baking dish. Top with cauliflower mix. Smooth out surface with a spoon. Cover with shredded cheddar cheese.
9) Bake 30 minutes, until cheese is melted and golden brown.

Nutrition Values

- Calories: 487
- Fat: 37g
- Carbohydrates: 11g
- Protein: 28g
- Dietary Fiber: 3.5g

57.Sweet and Sour Pork Chop

(Prep time: 5 minutes\ Cook time: 10 minutes| 4 servings)

Pork chops are sometimes a difficult dish to prepare as they are a dry meat. With this recipe, don't be afraid! You will create the perfect chop.

Ingredients:

For the recipe

- 4 pork chops, bone in
- 1 teaspoon of fine grain salt
- ⅛ teaspoon of fresh ground black pepper
- 2 Tablespoons of butter

For the glaze

- 2 Tablespoons of balsamic vinegar
- 2 Tablespoons of honey
- 2 garlic cloves, minced
- ½ teaspoon of dried rosemary
- ½ teaspoon of dried oregano
- Pinch of red pepper flakes

Preparation:

Preheat oven to 400F
1) Place a rack in the middle section.
2) Season the pork chops with salt and pepper. Set aside.
3) In a large iron skillet, melt the butter over medium-high heat.
4) While butter is sizzling, place the pork chops in the pan. Sear on both sides to create a crust. (Two minutes per side.)
5) Place the skillet in the oven, roast for 6 minutes.
6) As the meat cooks in the oven, in a saucepan, heat the balsamic vinegar, honey, garlic cloves, rosemary, oregano, red pepper flakes. Bring to a boil. Simmer to a thicker consistency.
7) Remove the skillet from the oven. Pour the sauce over the pork chops.
8) Return to the oven. Bake for 5 minutes.
9) Serve hot.

Nutrition Values

- Calories: 215
- Fat: 13g
- Carbohydrates: 11g
- Protein: 13g
- Dietary Fiber: 5g

58.Very Sweet Potatoes

Prep time: 15 minutes. Cook time: 35 minutes. Servings: 4.

Having being fed by our forefathers, sweet potatoes still remain in the clean eating platform.

Ingredients

- 4 sweet potatoes
- 1 tsp olive oil
- ½ tsp garlic salt
- ¼ tsp salt and fresh ground pepper

Preparation

Preheat oven to 400F

1. Wash the sweet potatoes. Slice thinly, with a knife or mandolin.
2. Rinse a few times under cold water.
3. Place slices in a large bowl. Drizzle olive oil, garlic powder, salt, and pepper over potato slices. Mix until evenly coated.
4. Spread slices in thin layer on parchment-covered baking sheets.
5. Bake potato slices 30 minutes, until crispy.

Nutrition Value

Calories: 114
Protein: 2.1g
Fat: 0.1g
Saturates: 0g
Carbs: 27g
Sugar: 6g
Fiber: 4g

59.Pumpkin Soup

Prep time: 15 minutes. Cook time: 45 minutes. Servings: 4.

Pumpkins are a rich source of vitamins, and in a soup you won't even notice you are eating healthy, it is that good!

Ingredients

- 2 Tbsp butter
- 1 small onion, diced
- 3 garlic cloves, minced
- ½ cup leeks, sliced
- 2 cups pumpkin puree
- 3 cups chicken broth
- 1 large carrot, minced
- 1 tsp fresh parsley
- ½ tsp fresh thyme
- ½ cup cooking cream
- ¼ tsp each salt and pepper

Preparation

1. In a large saucepan, melt the butter.
2. Sauté onion, garlic, leeks 4 minutes.
3. Add minced carrot. Cook 5 minutes. Stirring often.
4. Pour in pumpkin puree. Stir well.
5. Add chicken broth. Stir until fully combined.
6. Cover and cook 1 hour.
7. Using hand blender, emulsify the soup in the pot until a smooth consistency achieved.
8. Add the cream. Stir well. Serve hot.

Nutrition Value

Calories: 77
Protein: 2.51g
Fat: 2.5g
Saturates: 1.5g
Carbs: 11.03g
Sugar: 4.46g
Fiber: 3.1g

60.Stuffed Mushrooms

Prep time: 15 minutes. Cook time: 45 minutes. Servings: 2.

For a mushroom lover, few things in life can give more joy than this recipe.

Ingredients

- 1 pound mushrooms
- ½ cup (8 oz) Boursin cheese
- Paprika to garnish
- 1 Tbsp butter
- ¼ tsp garlic powder

Instructions

Preheat oven to 350F

1. Rinse mushrooms under cold water. Dry with paper towel. Gently remove the stems.
2. Mince the mushroom stems. In a small skillet, melt the butter. Add the stems. Season with garlic powder. Cook until tender. Spread them out on a plate to cool down slightly.
3. In a bowl, mash the Boursin cheese with a fork until soft. Mix in the cooked stems.
4. Fill mushroom caps with cheese mixture.
5. Place in a single layer on a parchment-covered baking sheet.
6. Season lightly with paprika.
7. Bake for 30 minutes, until caps tender. Serve hot.

Nutrition Value

Calories: 88
Protein: 2.7g
Fat: 8.2g
Saturates: 1g
Carbs: 1.5g
Sugar: 0g
Fiber: 0.5g

61.Lean Green Smoothie

Prep time: 15 minutes. Servings: 4.

Looking for an easy pick me up? Lean Green Smoothie!

Ingredients

- ¾ cup honeydew melon, peeled, diced
- 1 Tbsp ground angelica root
- ½ cup ice cubes
- 1 cup green seedless grapes
- 1 small cucumber, chopped
- ⅓ cup broccoli florets
- 1 sprig fresh mint

Directions

1. Place all ingredients in a blender.
2. Blend until smooth.
3. Pour in a glass. Serve immediately.

Nutrition Value

Calories: 133
Protein: 4.8g
Fat: 2g
Saturates: 1g
Carbs: 30.2g
Sugar: 23.7g
Fiber: 3.8g

62.Candied Pecans

(Prep time: 10 minutes\ Cook time: 60 minutes| 2 serving)

This sweet treat is sure to turn the head of any lover of nuts!

Ingredients:

- 2 cups of pecans
- 1 egg white
- 1 Tablespoon of water
- ¼ cup of honey
- Pinch of sea salt
- Pinch of cinnamon

Preparation:

Preheat oven to 250F
1) Cover a cookie sheet with parchment paper.
2) In a medium bowl, blend the egg white and water until fluffy.
3) Add the honey, cinnamon, and salt. Stir. Add pecans to the bowl. Stir until evenly coated.
4) Using a slotted spoon, transfer pecans in single layer to cookie sheet.
5) Bake for 60 minutes. Stir every 15 minutes.
6) Spread nuts on glass surface to cool.

Nutrition Values

Calories: 190 Fat: 17g Carbohydrates: 10g Protein: 1g; Dietary Fiber: 5g

63.Balsamic Rosemary Roasted Vegetables

(Prep time: 10 minutes\ Cook time: 60 minutes| 4 servings)

Whip up these rosemary coated vegetables for a kick to your immunity.

Ingredients:

- 2 cups of butternut squash, chopped in small cubes
- 1½ cups of broccoli florets
- ½ red onion, chopped in bite-size pieces
- 1 zucchini, chopped in bite-size pieces
- ½ red bell pepper, chopped in bite-size pieces
- 1 garlic clove, minced
- 2 Tablespoons of olive oil
- 1 Tablespoon of balsamic vinegar
- 1½ Tablespoons of fresh rosemary
- ½ Tablespoon of sea salt
- ½ teaspoon of black pepper

Preparation:

Preheat oven to 425F
1) Line a cookie sheet with parchment paper.
2) In a large bowl, whisk the vinegar, oil, salt and pepper.
3) Toss the vegetables in the oil until evenly coated.
4) Spread the mixture in a single layer on cookie sheet.
5) Bake for 45 - 60 minutes, until fork tender. Serve hot.

Nutrition Values

- Calories: 98
- Fat: 2.1g
- Carbohydrates: 19g
- Protein: 3g
- Dietary Fiber: 5g

64.Spiced and Crispy Carrot Chips

(Prep time: 50 minutes\ Cook time: 10 minutes| 1-2 servings)

Yes, you read that right. These paprika and cumin covered carrot chips might sound weird at first, but they are blast to have.

Ingredients:

- 3 cups of carrots sliced paper thin
- 2 Tablespoons of olive oil
- 2 teaspoons of ground cumin
- ½ teaspoon of smoked paprika
- Pinch of salt

Preparation:

Preheat oven to 400F
1) Cover a cookie sheet with parchment paper.
2) Using a sharp knife or mandolin, slice carrots paper thin.
3) In a large bowl, combine carrot slices with oil, cumin, paprika, and salt. Stir to evenly coat.
4) Place the pieces in a single layer on the cookie sheet.
5) Bake 8 - 10 minutes, until crispy.

65.Eggplant Caponata

(Prep time: 10 minutes\ Cook time: 20 minutes| 2 servings)

Another surprising recipe using an Eggplant, that leaves you fulfilled.

Ingredients:

- 2 Tablespoons of olive oil
- 3 garlic cloves, minced
- 2 onions, finely diced
- 4 cups of chopped eggplant
- 4 cups of chopped tomatoes
- 3 Tablespoons of white vinegar
- 2 Tablespoons of capers
- ½ cup of chopped up basil

Preparation:

1) In a large frying pan, drizzle oil over bottom of pan. Sauté the onions and garlic, until soft and translucent.
2) Cut up the eggplant. Add to the frying pan. Season with salt.
3) Cook eggplant 5 minutes, until fork tender. Drizzle oil over eggplant.
4) Add the tomatoes.
5) Stir in the vinegar.
6) Simmer 10 minutes, until the tomatoes are tender.
7) Serve in bowls. Garnish with basil and capers.

Nutrition Values

Calories: 175
Fat: 0g
Carbohydrates: 3g
Protein: 10g
Dietary Fiber: 5g

66.Sautéed Mushrooms

(Prep time: 10 minutes\ Cook time: 20 minutes| 2 servings)

Mushrooms...what can I say about Mushrooms? These are our favorite little fungi we love to eat! Yes, even as a snack.

Ingredients:

- 2 Tablespoons of butter
- 1 Tablespoon of olive oil
- 1½ pound of gourmet mushrooms
- 4 garlic cloves, diced
- ⅓ cup of white wine
- Pinch of salt

Preparation:

1) In a large, heavy skillet, heat up the oil and half the butter.
2) When the pan is almost smoking, add the mushrooms.
3) Stir the mushroom until soft and fork tender.
4) Add rest of the butter.
5) Stir in the garlic.
6) Add the white wine.
7) Once liquid has been absorbed, season with salt. Serve hot.

Nutrition Values

Calories: 124
Fat: 2g
Carbohydrates: 17g
Protein: 12g
Dietary Fiber: 0g

67.Sautéed Radishes
(Prep time: 5 minutes\ Cook time: 10 minutes| 6 servings)

You may be pleasantly surprised by experiencing this unique blend of multiple flavors from radishes.

Ingredients:

- 2 bunches of radishes, about 20 in total
- 1 Tablespoon of olive oil
- 1 teaspoon of butter
- 2 Tablespoons of honey
- 2 Tablespoons of white balsamic
- ¼ teaspoon of sea salt

Preparation:

Preheat oven to 350F
1) Slice the radishes to ¼ inch thickness.
2) In a large frying pan, heat the olive oil. Sauté the radishes.
3) Pour them into a baking dish.
4) In the same frying pan, melt the butter.
5) Add the honey. Stir in the balsamic vinegar and pinch of salt.
6) Pour the glaze over the radishes. Stir until evenly coated.
7) Heat the radishes in the oven for 15 minutes. Serve hot.

Nutrition Values

Calories: 25
Fat: 0.4g
Carbohydrates: 5g
Protein: 1g
Dietary Fiber: 2.4g

68.Roasted Heirloom Carrots

(Prep time: 10 minutes\ Cook time: 45 minutes| 3-4 servings)

These Roasted Heirloom carrots are crafted with the care they deserve for the taste buds that deserve them!

Ingredients:

- 1 bunch of fine heirloom carrots
- 1 Tablespoon of fresh thyme leaves
- ½ Tablespoon of coconut oil
- 1 Tablespoon of maple syrup
- ⅛ cup of freshly squeezed orange juices
- ⅛ teaspoon of sea salt

Preparation:

Preheat oven to 350F
1) Line a cookie sheet with parchment paper.
2) Thoroughly wash the carrots, remove any green parts.
3) In a small bowl, combine the coconut oil, maple syrup, orange juice, and sea salt. Stir until combined.
4) Pour mixture over carrots.
5) Spread the carrots out in a thin layer on the cookie sheet.
6) Sprinkle the carrots with thyme.
7) Roast for 45 minutes, or until fork tender.
8) Garnish with fresh thyme. Serve warm.

Nutrition Values

Calories: 70
Fat: 3g
Carbohydrates: 11g
Protein: 1g
Dietary Fiber: 3g

69.Beans With Crushed Almonds
(Prep time: 10 minutes\ Cook time: 20 minutes| 4 servings)

Get the health benefits of green beans in the form of a snack that is designed for a Paleo buff!

Ingredients:

- 1 pound of fresh green beans, ends trimmed
- 1½ Tablespoons of olive oil
- ¼ teaspoon of salt
- 1½ Tablespoons of fresh dill, minced
- Juice from 1 lemon
- ¼ cup of crushed almonds
- Sea salt for garnish

Preparation:

Preheat oven to 400F
1) Line a cookie sheet with parchment paper.
2) Toss green beans with olive oil. Season with salt.
3) Spread the green beans in a single layer across the cookie sheet.
4) Roast 10 minutes. Stir once.
5) Continue cooking for 8 – 10 minutes, until fork tender.
6) Remove from oven.
7) Place in a bowl. Drizzle lemon juice over the beans. Stir.
8) Garnish with fresh dill, crushed almonds, and sea salt.

Nutrition Values

Calories: 120
Fat: 8g
Carbohydrates: 13g
Protein: 4g
Dietary Fiber: 5g

70.Cauliflower Couscous with Apricots and Cashews

(Prep time: 20 minutes\ Cook time: 20 minutes| 4-6 servings)

Don't judge it before you taste it, as it just might turn out to be one of your favorite dishes.

Ingredients:

- 2 heads of cauliflower, diced in florets
- ½ cup of roasted cashew nut
- ⅓ cup of apricots, cut into raisin-size pieces
- 4 scallions, finely chopped
- 4 Tablespoons of fresh parsley, chopped
- 2 Tablespoons of fresh cilantro, chopped
- ¼ teaspoon of red pepper flakes
- Pinch of salt and pepper

For the Dressing

- 2 Tablespoons of dates, mashed
- 2 Tablespoons of olive oil
- 2 Tablespoons of water
- 1 Tablespoon of fresh lemon juice
- 2 Tablespoons of fresh orange juice
- 2 teaspoons of fresh ginger, grated
- ½ teaspoon of ground cinnamon
- Pinch of salt and pepper

Preparation:

Preheat oven to 425F
1) Drizzle oil lightly over large baking sheet.
2) Place the cauliflower florets in a food processor. Pulse until a rice-like consistency is achieved.
3) Spread out the cauliflower in a thin layer on the baking sheet.
4) Bake for 15-20 minutes, stirring every 5 minutes.
5) Remove from oven. Allow to cool completely.
6) Mash the dates using a food processor.
7) Dressing: In a large bowl, combine the mashed dates, olive oil, water, lemon juice, orange juice, ginger, cinnamon, salt, and pepper. Whisk to combine.
8) Pour in the cooled cauliflower. Stir until evenly coated with dressing. Serve.

Nutrition Values

- Calories: 570
- Fat: 21g
- Carbohydrates: 25g
- Protein: 17g
- Dietary Fiber: 6.3g

CHAPTER 6: MEAL PREP FOR SWEET TREATS

71.Flourless Chocolate Cake

Prep time: 15 minutes. Cook time: 50 minutes. Servings: 10.

Sugar-free, gluten-free, dairy-free, grain-free, corn-free, soy-free, and paleo... could it still be delicious? But, of course!

Ingredients

- 1½ cups packed pitted dates
- 1½ cups packed almond meal
- ½ tsp baking soda
- ½ cup cocoa powder
- 3 eggs
- 2 tsp vanilla
- ½ cup water
- 2 Tbsp coconut oil
- pinch of salt

Preparation

Preheat oven to 325F

1. In a medium bowl, combine almond meal, baking soda, cocoa powder, salt.
2. In a separate bowl, blend water and dates. Stir until a paste forms. Mix in eggs, vanilla, and coconut oil.
3. Combine wet and dry ingredients. Stir until smooth.
4. Pour batter into a round, flavorless oiled cake pan.
5. Bake 30 minutes.
6. Cool 15 minutes before serving.

Nutrition Value

Calories: 10
Protein: 4g
Fat: 15g
Saturates: 0g
Carbs: 15g
Sugar: 7g
Fiber: 0g

72. Biscotti with Almonds

Prep time: 15 minutes. Cook time: 50 minutes. Servings: 2.

These biscotti with almonds possess all the necessary qualities of something sweet to soak in your tea or coffee.

Ingredients:

- sugar substitute
- ½ cup butter, room temperature
- 2 eggs, room temperature
- 3 cups almond meal
- ¼ teaspoon salt
- 1 tablespoon baking powder
- 1 tsp vanilla extract
- 2 tsp almond extract
- ½ cup slivered almonds

Preparation:

Preheat oven to 350F

1. In a medium bowl, combine sugar substitute and butter. Beat until combined.
2. Add one egg at a time to combined sugar mixture. Beat until combined. Add vanilla extract. Stir. Add almond extract. Stir.
3. In a separate bowl, combine almond meal, salt, baking powder. Stir.
4. Combine dry ingredients with wet ingredients. Stir gently.
5. Let batter rest 5 minutes. Pour onto parchment-lined cookie sheet. Spread almond slices over top of batter in a thin layer.
6. Bake 25 minutes. Remove pan from oven. Cool 10 minutes.
7. Cut into slices.
8. Place cookies sideways on cookie sheet.
9. Bake additional 15 minutes. Cool 5 minutes.

Nutrition Value

Calories: 70
Protein: 1.4g
Fat: 3.2g
Saturates: 1g
Carbs: 0.7g
Sugar: 4.2g
Fiber: 1g

73.Strawberry Yogurt Cornflake Parfait

Prep time: 15 minutes. Servings: 4.

An easy way for a sweet treat!

Ingredients

- 1 tub strawberry-flavored yogurt
- 2 kiwis, peeled, sliced
- 2 Tbsp cornflakes natures
- 4 fresh strawberries, sliced
- Few drops lemon juice
- Mint leaves

Preparation

1. In a medium bowl, mix the strawberries and kiwi with lemon juice.
2. In a clear glass, spoon a layer of yogurt along bottom.
3. Spread a layer of strawberries over yogurt.
4. Spoon in layer of yogurt over strawberries.
5. Spread a layer of kiwi over yogurt.
6. Spread a layer of yogurt over kiwi slices.
7. Spoon in layer of yogurt.
8. Spread strawberries over yogurt.
9. Spread a layer of yogurt over strawberries. Top with cornflakes. Garnish with mint leaves.

Nutrition Value

Calories: 170
Protein: 4g
Fat: 3g
Saturates: 2g
Carbs: 33g
Sugar: 20g
Fiber: 1g

74.Choco Berry Mousse

Prep time: 15 minutes Cook time: 20 minutes. Servings: 2.

Chocolate and raspberry are two flavors that blend blissfully together.

Ingredients
- 6 raspberries
- ⅓ cup heavy whipping cream
- 4 Drops liquid sweetener
- 1 tsp unsweetened cocoa powder
- 1 Tbsp chocolate whey powder
- 1 Tbsp dark chocolate flakes

Preparation
1. In a large mixing bowl, blend the cream until stiff peaks form. Add 2 drops of sweetener. Stir. (Taste it. Add more sweetener if needed.)
2. Stir in cocoa powder, whey powder, and flakes. Whisk until blended and smooth.
3. Chill 1 hour before serving. Garnish with fresh raspberries.

Nutrition Value
Calories: 330
Protein: 10g
Fat: 33g
Saturates: 2g
Carbs: 12g
Sugar: 1g
Fiber: 0.5g

75.Strawberry Frozen Yogurt

Prep time: 15 minutes. Servings: 4.

A sweet treat sure to fill any fussy palette.

Ingredients

- 3 cups frozen strawberries
- ½ cup granulated Splenda
- ½ cup non-fat plain yogurt
- 1 Tbsp lemon juice

Preparation

1. In a food processor, combine strawberries, Splenda. Pulse until fruit chopped up.
2. Add the lemon juice, pulse again.
3. Add the yogurt. Pulse again until smooth.
4. Place in freezer. Chill 2 hours. Use ice cream scooper to portion.

76.Avocado Smoothie

Prep time: 15 minutes. Servings: 4.

Avocado smoothie is the best snack for a weight loss enthusiast.

Ingredients

- ½ avocado, diced
- ¼ cup coconut milk
- ¼ cup fresh baby spinach
- ¼ cup fresh mint
- 1 tsp cinnamon
- 2 Tbsp pistachio nuts
- 1 tsp vanilla extract
- 5 drops liquid Stevia
- Ice cubes

Preparation
1. Make sure to rinse the mint leaves and spinach leaves. Dice up the avocado.
2. Place all the ingredients in a blender.
3. Add a few ice cubes at first, to test consistency.
4. Blend until smooth. Serve immediately.

Nutrition Value

Calories: 200.99
Protein: 4.03g
Fat: 17.26g
Saturates: 7.05g
Carbs: 10.62g
Sugar: 1.92g
Fiber: 5.46g

77.Raspberry-Peach Crumble

Prep time: 10 minutes. Cook time: 30 minutes. Servings: 8.

An old-fashioned favorite.

Ingredients
Crumble Topping
- ¾ cup healthy flour
- ¼ cup sugar substitute
- ¼ packed brown sugar
- ¾ teaspoon cinnamon
- ¼ cup chopped walnuts or pecans
- 6 Tbsp melted butter

Filling
- ¼ cup sugar substitute
- 2 teaspoons cornstarch
- 9 fresh peaches, peeled and sliced
- 1 cup fresh raspberries

Preparation
Preheat oven to 375F
1. Crumble: In a medium bowl, whisk together flour, sugar substitute, and cinnamon. Add melted butter and mix. Set aside.
2. Filling: In a small bowl, whisk together sugar substitute and cornstarch. Set side.
3. Using a 3-4 quart baking dish, add sliced peaches and raspberries. Spread cornstarch mixture over peaches. Stir to coat evenly.
4. Sprinkle crumble topping over peaches and raspberries.
5. Place baking dish on a cookie sheet. Bake 30 minutes, or until topping is golden brown and peaches are fork tender.
6. Serve warm.

Nutrition Value
Calories: 327
Protein: 2.5g
Fat: 16.5g
Saturates: 2g
Carbs: 44.3g
Sugar: 3g
Fiber: 1g

78.Fresh Strawberry Parfait

Prep time: 20 minutes. Servings: 4.

Finish your dinner with this sweet and light dessert.

Ingredients
- 4 cups fresh strawberries, sliced
- 1 cup fat-free ricotta cheese
- 4 ounces low-fat cream cheese, room temperature
- ½ cup granulated sugar substitute
- 8 amaretto cookies, crushed
- 1 tsp vanilla
- 4 Tbsp almond slivers

Preparation
1. Using a blender, puree 2 cups strawberries and ¼ cup sugar substitute. Remove to a bowl and set aside.
2. In a medium bowl, blend the ricotta cheese, cream cheese, ¼ cup sugar substitute, and vanilla. Add a little water if mixture is too thick.
3. Use 4 parfait glasses, assemble parfaits:
4. Spoon in 2 tablespoons crushed cookies in bottom of each glass.
5. Spoon in 2 tablespoons strawberry puree.
6. Spoon in layer sliced strawberries.
7. Spoon in layer cream cheese mixture. Repeat until glasses are filled.
8. Top with almond slivers. Chill for 30 minutes then serve.

Nutrition Value
Calories: 215
Protein: 17g
Fat: 2g
Saturates: 0g
Carbs: 34g
Sugar: 8g
Fiber: 5g

79.Beets & Berries Smoothie

Prep time: 20 minutes. Servings: 4.

A sweet treat you won't know is good for you!

Ingredients
- ¼ cup coconut yogurt
- 1 cup fresh blueberries
- ½ cup fresh raspberries
- ⅓ cup beets, sliced
- ¼ cup orange juice
- 1 tsp honey
- 1 Tbsp vanilla protein powder
- 1 Tbsp chia seeds (optional)
- 1 cup ice cubes
- ½ cup lettuce leaves

Preparation
1. In a blender, combine all the ingredients. Blend until smooth.
2. Serve immediately.

Nutrition Value
Calories: 120.97
Protein: 2.56g
Fat: 2.27g
Saturates: 0.22g
Carbs: 25.96g
Sugar: 15.7g
Fiber: 6.72g

80.Strawberry Cheesecake

Prep time: 25 minutes. Cook time: 60 minutes. Servings: 8.

Cheesecake can be part of a diet plan!

Ingredients
Crust

- ½ cup Pecans
- ¾ Cup of Almond Flour
- 4 Tablespoons of Butter
- 2 Tablespoons of Sweetener

Filling

- 2 x 8 oz cream cheese, room temperature
- ¼ cup sour cream, room temperature
- 4 Eggs, room temperature
- ½ Tbsp Lemon Juice, room temperature
- ½ Tbsp pure vanilla extract
- 9 - 15 Strawberries

Preparation
Preheat oven to 400F

Crust

1. Crush Pecans. Combine pecans, flour, and sweetener.
2. Melt butter. Combine butter with pecan mixture.
3. Press crumb mixture into spring-form pan.
4. Bake 5 minutes, until golden brown. Set aside to cool.

Filling

1. In a large bowl, blend the cream cheese until smooth.
2. Stir in sour cream. Add one egg at a time. Stir until combined. Add lemon juice. Stir. Add vanilla. Stir.
3. Dice up 5 strawberries, add to batter. Stir until ingredients combined.
4. Slice rest of strawberries in half. Line against spring-form pan, above crust.
5. Pour in cheesecake batter.
6. Bake 55 minutes.
7. Cool completely. Refrigerate 3 hours before slicing.
8. Garnish with fresh strawberries and cream.

Nutrition Value
Calories: 535

Protein: 13g

Fat: 49g

Saturates: 1g

Carbs: 9g

Sugar: 0g

Fiber: 1.75g

81. Fruit Granita

Prep Time: 30 minutes. Ready in: 5 hours. Servings: 2.

This fruit granita uses fresh fruit to sweeten the pot.

Ingredients

- 1 cup fresh raspberries
- 1 cup fresh blueberries
- 1 cup unsweetened apple juice
- ¼ cup fresh lime juice
- 4 cups cubed ripe melon
- Fresh mint leaves, for garnish

Preparation

1. Start with combining the apple juice, melon and lime juice. Blend until smooth. Pour into metal or glass pan.
2. Freeze the pan, scraping and stirring with a fork every half hour until the granita is hard, approximately 3-4 hours.
3. Next, remove the granite from the freezer and break it up into small pieces. Freeze again for 1 hour.
4. Serve in glass dishes. Garnish with fresh mint leaves.

Nutrition Value

Calories: 70
Protein: 1g
Fat: 1g
Saturates: 1g
Carbs: 17g
Sugar: 0g
Fiber: 0g

82.Graham Crackers

(Prep time: 15 minutes| Cook time: 30 minutes| 4-6 servings)

Sometimes you feel like a snack, sometimes you don't. This graham cracker cookie can fulfill you until a next meal, and they are perfect for Paleo Diet.

Ingredients:

- 2¼ cups full almond flour
- 1 teaspoon of baking powder
- 1 teaspoon of ground cinnamon
- ½ teaspoon of fine sea salt
- 1 large egg
- 2 Tablespoons of melted coconut oil
- 2 Tablespoons of pure maple syrup

Preparation:

1) In a large bowl, whisk the dry ingredients together; almond flour, baking powder, cinnamon, and sea salt.
2) In a separate bowl, combine the egg, maple syrup, and coconut oil together. Stir until blended.
3) Pour the wet mixture into the dry ingredients. Stir until a dough forms and pulls away from the sides.
4) Cover with plastic wrap. Chill the dough for 30 minutes.
5) Preheat oven to temperature 325F. Cover a large cookie sheet with parchment paper.
6) Roll out the dough to ⅛ inch thickness.
7) Using a pizza cutter or sharp knife, cut out 2.5 inch squares, transfer to cookie sheet.
8) Bake 15 minutes, until golden brown.
9) Cool 5 minutes before removing from cookie sheet.

83.Mango Chia Seed Pudding

(Prep time: 10 minutes\ Cook time: 60 minutes| 4 servings)

This double layer pudding will satisfy any hunger.

Ingredients:

- 3 Tablespoons of chia seeds
- 1 cup of vanilla coconut milk or almond milk
- 2 Tablespoons maple syrup
- Pinch of cinnamon
- Pinch of cardamom
- 1 teaspoon pure vanilla extract
- 1 mango, peeled, pureed

Preparation:

1) In a medium bowl with an air tight lid, combine the chia seeds, milk (coconut or almond), 1 tablespoon of the maple syrup, cinnamon, and cardamom.
2) Whisk the ingredients until combined. Place air tight lid on mixture. Refrigerate 8 – 12 hours.
3) When ready to serve. Prepare the mango: puree the mango in a food processor. Pour into a bowl. Add 1 tablespoon of maple syrup. Stir until combined. You could chill it briefly.
4) Using clear jars, alternate layers of chia pudding and mango puree. Serve immediately or refrigerate until ready to eat.

Nutrition Values

- Calories: 146
- Fat: 26g
- Carbohydrates: 15g
- Protein: 23g
- Dietary Fiber: 11.2g

84.Chocolaty Cocoa Mousse

(Prep time: 10 minutes\ Cook time: nil| 4 servings)

In just a few minutes, you can whip up a batch of this fine mousse.

Ingredients:

- Coconut cream scraped from upper side of 2 x 13.5 ounce cans chilled of full fat coconut milk
- 4 Tablespoons of cocoa
- 3 Tablespoons of honey
- 1 teaspoon of pure vanilla extract

Preparation:

1) The first step is to open the chilled cans of coconut milk and scoop out the thick cream. Place in a large bowl.
2) To that bowl, add the honey, cocoa, pure vanilla extract. Beat using your mixer, start low to medium until a nice foam appears.
3) Divide the mixture evenly into ramekins. Chill 30 to 60 minutes.

Nutrition Values

Calories: 134 Fat: 3.8g Carbohydrates: 16g Protein: 3.8g Dietary Fiber: 8.1g

85.Pumpkin Nut Butter Cup

(Prep time: 120 minutes\ Cook time: nil| 4 servings)

Who says muffins are banned on Paleo? This recipe will allow you to create exquisitely delicious pumpkin nut butter cups with multiple layers of goodness.

Ingredients:

For Filing

- ½ cup of organic pumpkin puree
- ½ cup of homemade almond butter
- 2 Tablespoons of organic maple syrup
- 4 Tablespoons of organic coconut oil
- ¼ teaspoon of organic ground nutmeg
- ¼ teaspoon of organic ground ginger
- 1 teaspoon of organic ground cinnamon
- ⅛ teaspoon of organic ground clove
- 2 teaspoons of pure vanilla extract

For Topping

- 1 cup of organic raw cacao powder
- 4 Tablespoons of organic maple syrup
- 1 cup of organic coconut oil

Preparation:

1) In a large mixing bowl, combine the pumpkin puree, almond butter, maple syrup, nutmeg, ginger, cinnamon, cloves, and vanilla extract. Blend on low to medium until smooth and creamy.
2) In another bowl, combine the cacao powder, maple syrup, coconut oil. Blend from low to medium until smooth and creamy.
3) Fill a muffin tin with paper liners. Fill the liners ⅓ full with chocolate filling. Place in freezer for 15 minutes.
4) Pour a layer ⅓ with pumpkin filling. Return to freezer for 15 minutes.
5) Pour top layer ⅓ of chocolate mix. Place in freezer. Chill for 2 hours.

Nutrition Values

- Calories: 105
- Fat: 10.1g
- Carbohydrates: 3.3g
- Protein: 2.9g
- Dietary Fiber: 1.3g

86.Chocolate Silk Pie

(Prep time: 90 minutes\ Cook time: 10 minutes| 16 servings)

This is a fairly simple recipe that will teach you how to bake up your very own chocolate silk pie. A delightful layer of chocolate mousse that is mixed with a healthy boost of avocados.

Ingredients:

Crust:

- 28 Chocolate cookie wafers
- 2 Tablespoons sugar
- 4 Tablespoons unsalted butter, melted
- Pinch of salt

Filling:

- 8 ounces of Dark Chocolate
- ¼ cup of extra virgin olive oil
- 2 ripe Avocados
- 1 cup of coconut sugar
- 1½ cups of cocoa powder
- 1 cup of heavy cream
- 1 Tablespoon of vanilla
- ½ teaspoon of espresso powder
- Pinch of salt

Preparation:

Crust:

Preheat oven to 350F

1) Pulse the wafers, sugar, salt in food processor until you have a crumbly, sandy mixture. Add melted butter. Pulse lightly to combine.
2) Pour into a 9-inch pie pan. Press firmly on crumb mixture along bottom and up sides of pie dish. Bake for 10 minutes. Allow to cool completely before filling.

Filling:

1) Melt the dark chocolate; using double-boiler method or microwave. Stir in coconut oil. Set aside. Cool to room temperature.
2) Scoop out avocado meat. Place in a mixing bowl. Mash the avocado completely until smooth.
3) Add the chocolate mixture to bowl with avocado. Whip for 1-2 minutes with electric mixer, until smooth consistency.
4) Stir in the cocoa powder and sugar. Whip 1 minute, until smooth.
5) Add the vanilla extract, cream, salt, and espresso. Whip again until smooth and fluffy, approximately 2 minutes.
6) Pour the batter over pie crust. Chill for 2 hours.
7) Serve with whipped cream!

Nutrition Values

- Calories: 265
- Fat: 4g
- Carbohydrates: 12g
- Protein: 1g
- Dietary Fiber: 1g

87.Cinnamon Apple Chips

(Prep time: 10 minutes\ Cook time: 120 minutes| 4 servings)

We don't really consider apples as anything but a healthy snack. Well, now, you can have your chips and eat 'em, too!

Ingredients:

- 2 organic apples
- Cinnamon

Preparation:

Preheat oven to 225F
1) Using a sharp knife or mandolin, slice the apples thinly.
2) Line cookie sheet with parchment paper. Arrange slices in single layer. Lightly sprinkle cinnamon over the slices.
3) Bake for an hour. Flip the slices over. Sprinkle a light layer of cinnamon over apple slices. Bake for another hour. (Apples should no longer moist by end of baking.)
4) Remove the chips. Cool for 10 minutes before eating.
5) Store in air tight container.

Nutrition Values

Calories: 175 Fat: 36g Carbohydrates: 16g Protein: 12g Dietary Fiber: 10g

88. Blueberry Smoothie

(Prep time: 10 minutes\ Cook time: 120 minutes| 10 ounce)

This blend is nothing short of Popeye's very own power-enhancing mixture!

Ingredients:

- ½ a frozen banana
- ¾ cup of frozen blueberries
- 1 handful of spinach leaves
- ¾ cup of nonfat honey Greek yogurt
- ⅔ cup of almond coconut milk
- 1 Tablespoon of hemp hearts
- 1 Tablespoon of vanilla whey protein powder
- 1 teaspoon of maca powder
- 1 teaspoon of maple syrup
- Bee pollen

Preparation:

1) Place all the ingredients in a blender. Pulse until smooth.
2) Chill 15 minutes to 2 hours. Enjoy!

Nutrition Values

Calories: 261 Fat: 4.2g Carbohydrates: 20g Protein: 10.1g Dietary Fiber: 4.6g

Conclusion

As for meal prep, it is well worth experimenting, and finding the snacks, drinks, and meals that fit best with your palette. These recipes are nutritional and come with many health benefits. These weight loss recipes also have a distinct flavor and tastes that make them enjoyable, even on a diet. Hope you enjoyed them!

Thank you for purchasing this book. I hope this book has been of great importance to you and set to start out the meal prepping.